Breath in Action

of related interest

Vital Breath of the Dao
Chinese Shamanic Tiger Qigong – Laohu Gong
Master Zhongxian Wu
ISBN 978 1 84819 000 9

Meet Your Body
A Rolfer's Guide to Releasing Bodymindcore Trauma
Noah Karrasch
Illustrated by Lovella Lindsey
ISBN 978 1 84819 016 0

Experiential Chi Kung
You Are How You Move
Ged Sumner
ISBN 978 1 84819 014 6

Breath in Action

The Art of Breath in Vocal and Holistic Practice

EDITED BY JANE BOSTON
AND RENA COOK

FOREWORD BY CICELY BERRY

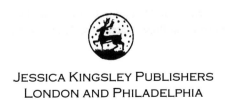

JESSICA KINGSLEY PUBLISHERS
LONDON AND PHILADELPHIA

First published in 2009
by Jessica Kingsley Publishers
116 Pentonville Road
London N1 9JB, UK
and
400 Market Street, Suite 400
Philadelphia, PA 19106, USA

www.jkp.com

Library of Congress Cataloging in Publication Data
Breath in action : the art of breath in vocal and holistic practice / edited by Jane Boston and Rena Cook.
p. cm.
ISBN 978-1-84310-942-6 (pb : alk. paper) 1. Respiration. 2. Voice culture. 3. Breathing exercises. I. Boston, Jane. II. Cook, Rena.
RA782.B74 2009
613'.192--dc22

2008052200

British Library Cataloguing in Publication Data
A CIP catalogue record for this book is available from the British Library

ISBN 978 1 84310 942 6

Dedications

For Joe
Rena Cook

For Liz, my mother, who knew a thing or two about the breath of life
Jane Boston

Acknowledgements

Many people assisted and supported us in the five years of this project. I say a heart felt thank you to:

Past and present students in the School of Drama at the University of Oklahoma who inspired me to dig deeper including Eudaemone Jervis Battilega, Amy Vorphal, Steven Knight, Marlowe Holden, Amy Brown, Dana McConnell and Walter Elder; administrators and colleagues including Tom Houston Orr, Marvin Lamb, Eugene Enrico, Kae Koger and Sheila Rinear.

Rena Cook

To Siren Theatre for revealing how theatre works and why it matters.

My colleagues at the Royal Academy of Dramatic Art for deepening the discussion. My family for their abiding loyalty, especially my father for his editorial and journalistic expertize and Ella for being herself.

To Jac for the integrity of her thoughts on life, her capacity to feel, her take on what is and for the fact that her dreams about what might be stand a great chance of coming true.

Jane Boston

To our assistant Cassidy Elms who organized us and read every word of this book—more than once.

Contents

Foreword

I was delighted to be asked to write the foreword to this book for I believe it to be extremely important in that it brings together the views and beliefs of so many voice, holistic, alternative health and movement practitioners, each of whom have their own very specific way of viewing the place of breath in their practice. This collection will dispel some of the mystery, which I think builds up once we start talking about 'methods'. From my own standpoint as a theatre voice practitioner, it has enabled me to catch up on the many new and different approaches in the way we think about breath – our perception of both its artistic and its technical values – its inspiration in other words! And this has made me look for a moment at my own specific journey in relation to training actors and an approach to breath and how in the process so much has changed.

Training at the Central School of Speech and Drama between 1943 and 1946 under the direction of the wonderful Gwynneth Thurburn, I was reared on 'rib reserve'. This involved opening out the ribs, separating the rib movement from that of the diaphragm, so that the chest was enlarged both by widening and by deepening the movement of the lungs. This gave the voice a strong chest resonance, while we spoke on the diaphragm breath. It was all physically demanding and I often found it to be over-technical and difficult. However, it was the method taught when, in 1948, I went back to teach there full-time on the actor training programme.

Over time, the great thing I got out of my work at Central was the focus put on the speaking of verse, both classical and modern – something in which Gwynneth put great store and which fulfilled my own passion and need for poetry. For me breath has always been about fulfilling the thought and the word.

It was not until 1970, when Trevor Nunn invited me to join the Royal Shakespeare Company that I began consciously to think about the breath in a different way. Initially my job at the RSC was to ensure that the actors could reach the perimeters of the auditorium with clarity and without vocal strain. But as I began to work more closely with the directors at the time, my focus became helping the individual actors maintain their own vocal truth whilst also fulfilling the demands of the space and the demands of those directors, each of whom had very different styles. The focus was then on the text.

My beginning at the RSC also coincided with the time when styles of acting began to change. We no longer wanted to hear that well-rounded, 'poetic' sound for it was no longer relevant; television was in our ears and we wanted to hear real people speaking. We wanted to hear the actor's own personal truth. And it was at this point that I found the whole concept of rib reserve no longer useful. It was too much aligned to the technical constraints of singing, of fulfilling a time frame or phrase, of finding music within the phraseology. It was clearly not about finding and discovering the thought itself.

The voice is the actor's principal means of communication, of exciting the audience and with the text and the ideas contained therein, of provoking a response and of making a change. Underneath it all is the breath. We, as audience, want the actor to draw us into their thoughts, their world, their imaginings, to find the words within themselves – I like to call it 'sitting down in the voice'. To do this, the actor needs to be in charge of their own voice so that it is as open and free as possible, both in tone and pitch. So my focus regarding breath is as follows:

- regular breathing exercises with the ribs to open out the chest without tension, so that the speaker/actor is conscious of their own resonance in the body

- working on language/text with the diaphragm breath, feeling that breath settle inside as deeply as possible, thus being aware of sound and thought starting from the centre

- becoming aware of resonance in one's seat – so that the resonance/vibration is felt throughout the body.

In these ways, the listener is drawn by the true resonance in the speaker's voice.

I do believe the actor today has a difficult job whether working on classical or modern text. If classical, the need is to make it sound as if it is being spoken now, whilst at the same time fulfilling and conveying the size of the language, the size of the feelings – the 'earth-shifts' as Edward Bond would call them – fully to the hearer, which is a continual balancing act. And conversely, when working on modern text, the need is to embody the private and intimate feelings which are there and to convey those feelings simply, while finding the precision of the words so that the underlying subtext lands with precision on the hearer. And for this to happen, we rely on our breath – the breath is the thought. This has been my own journey.

In this book, Rena Cook and Jane Boston have brought together a remarkable collection of writing from so many diverse practitioners, all prestigious and all with their own beliefs and experiences of the working of the breath. It will be of great value to all those who work with health-giving holistic practices and the arts of communication.

Cicely Berry, OBE Hon. D. Lit

Voice Director: Royal Shakespeare Company

Introduction

JANE BOSTON AND RENA COOK

Breath *is* life. Breath is key to all human activity. Breath is essential to survival. We breathe or we die. Yet breath is rarely examined in detail.

At a rate of approximately eighteen times per minute, one thousand and eighty times an hour and twenty-five thousand nine hundred and twenty times a day, it is not surprising there is a desire to ignore this complex, repetitive activity. Clearly, to be conscious of it at all times would be unbearable. Equally, however, to remain oblivious is to ignore the possibility that changing the awareness and use of the breath can make a radical difference to human functioning, particularly to an individual's ability to express her or himself.

Breath provides an essential key not just to our being but also to our communicative function. Once we admit breath into consciousness we become aware that it is no longer just a psycho-physical phenomenon, but is also subject to social and cultural values. The conscious use and subsequent management of breath, therefore, whether in the areas of health improvement, holistic practice or performance, begins the process towards creative and health-giving enhancement. The head of alternative medicine at the University of Arizona highlights this possibility: 'When people ask me what single lifestyle change has the greatest potential for promoting good health, my answer is: Learn how to breathe correctly' (Weil 1999, p. 5).

With each new generation of teacher and student, the traditions underpinning breath work in health, holistic or performance practice require investigation if they are to remain relevant. Since the advances of science, changing social norms and shifting aesthetics all play a role in the construction of existing practices, the integration of new knowledge is essential towards the creation of more effective teaching and learning techniques.

In this book, a group of leading contemporary practitioners and theorists from the arts, the healing arts and the speech and medical sciences examines the similarities and divergences that arise out of their traditions. They do this in order to create a robust, multi-voiced discourse about the science, theory and the practice of breath.

The shared authorship enables the range, subtlety and profundity of the subject to be fully covered, reflecting the editors' wish that the understanding, pedagogy and practice relating to breath for human communication be examined in its widest possible sense. In order to fully address this, the interdisciplinary focus of the book is designed to generate a creative cross-fertilization between the research and practices of various subject areas in which breath occupies a key position. It is hoped that this will not only contribute to the development of a wider understanding of the breath in action, but also to its application in a number of communicative and holistic fields.

Who, then, will benefit from this close examination of breath? The performer on stage, the teacher with their students, the patient seeking a holistic medical cure, the alternative health practitioner and the lawyer in court are all linked by their desire to be healthy and to communicate effectively. The thin, querulous voice and ungrounded body of the unsupported performer, the constricted speech of the teacher, the shallow breath of the ailing patient, the inaudibility of the lawyer all share the common challenge of breath as it inhibits successful communication.

We can also see in all these examples a display of physical symptoms that indicate an imbalance in the means of communication that is not just inefficient but also unhealthy. The desire to make a meaningful connection with an audience, to hold a classroom in rapt attention, to rediscover health and vigour, or to win a favourable verdict, are all destabilized and impeded by the lack of appropriate breath.

Although on the one hand these examples are clearly representative of very different applications of the breath, they all demonstrate the key importance of breath awareness to positive transformation of all kinds. They also demonstrate the extent to which the practice background of many of the books' contributors in the area of vocal studies, has long provided the unifying focus of voice, mind, body and breath in a way that is also consistent with wider holistic practice.

The enquiry begins with the anatomy and physiology of breath and provides an unequivocal starting point from which all investigations of theory and practice can depart and return. Here, the authors document important instances of the ways in which the knowledge of the multiple physical systems that relate to breath can provide real opportunities for a dialogue between the medical sciences, alternative health care practitioners and performance practitioners.

In a macro sense, the research and practice about breath has demonstrated that performances improve, health flourishes, audiences engage and individuals develop professional longevity. At a micro level, where insightful and nuanced pedagogy is championed, the relationships between breath and the word, for example, have been proven to produce a detailed and profound enrichment of the smallest moments of theatrical craft and the patterns of movement of the diaphragm have been shown to link very directly with the expression of human emotion (Nakamura 1981, p.15).

Public speaking, for example, is enhanced as an activity when work on the breath contributes to the training processes of the individuals involved. Organic dance forms can flourish, new spectatorships encouraged and movement practitioners can create more sustainable and uniquely defined careers when breath is attended to. The arts of both acting and singing, with their requirements of refined utterance and healthy management, are enhanced in multiple ways if the training pedagogies have breath at their core. And finally, all those can be helped who are involved in the public arts of litigation and political persuasion, or the healing arts of medical and alternative therapies, where breath is crucial to both success and healing:

> Regular diaphragm movements stimulate the solar plexus and stabilize the mental functions. This in turn results in a stabilization of the respiration cycle and a consequent stabilization of and improvement in mental and physical condition (Nakamura 1981, p.28).

Breath, in all these contexts, can be a fruitful diagnostic tool by which the perceptions of entrenched habit and communicative imbalances can be assessed and remedial action taken. It can also be the means of transformation for an individual in both performance and life, as their weaknesses and strengths are revealed and confronted through the medium of the breath.

Clearly breath can be both an effective tool to diagnose and to generate change. It is also symbolic of the possibilities of change and as such is integrated in much of the philosophical aspects of the writing in the book. In particular, the frequently documented split in thought and practice between East and West features profoundly. Here breath provides the very specific pivot in the West upon which much desired change of perspective and habit hinges.

The contemporary climate also provides its own imperative for a deeper under-standing of breath. A well-documented cultural move away from all processes that involve time, personal investment and deep analysis, toward those that offer a sense of immediate gratification provides another strong impulse for many authors. There is much argument put forth by those who support the idea of breath as an ingredient in enabling artistic freedom alongside those who make a case for breath in its role in preventative medical practice, the process of which takes time to bear fruit. By ex-ploring the reasons underpinning a cultural phenomenon of 'haste', the authors offer ways to enable these trends to be understood and reveal practices that allow them to be reconfigured.

By both reflecting debate and provoking new thinking, this book offers a col-lective voice of expertise to provide an advanced student and practitioner guide to current thinking and trends in the field of training in breath, health and voice. It provides new rationales based on current theory and practice and suggests new ways of working in the light of relevant thinking, whether you are involved as a trainer in creating programmes within these fields or simply as an individual wishing to en-hance your own ability and understanding.

Organized with four subject headings to highlight the specific scholarship and practices pertaining to those areas, plurality of style is also a conscious aspect of the design and content of the book. The mix of personal narrative, historical scholar-ship and practice-based evidence offers a dynamic and productive eclecticism for the reader in order to better access and understand the potency, impact and authority of the breath.

The starting point has been provided by the microcosmic example of breath within a range of performance and body mind contexts, but all the principles and techniques explored clearly inform the macrocosm of human existence at all levels. In subtle and profound ways, breath supports, clarifies and intensifies not only all human communication but also a healthy response to survival in a rich, complex and challenging world.

BIBLIOGRAPHY

Nakamura, Takashi (1981) *Oriental Breathing Therapy.* Tokyo and New York: Japan Publications.

Weil, A. (1999) *Breathing: The Master Key to Self Healing.* Massachusetts: Thorne Communications.

SECTION 1

Breath and the Body

JANE BOSTON AND RENA COOK

The opening chapters of this interdisciplinary dialogue between medical scientists, alternative health, voice and holistic practitioners, take the subject of the body for their focus. This structure is designed both to provide a common and irrefutable starting point for subsequent enquiry and also to foster meaningful communicative pathways between a range of disciplines, where cross referring the evidences of science and experiential practices can lead to more effective change.

The theorization of the breath in the body offered in neuromuscular, medical and speech sciences models begins this process. Collectively, they provide an important foundational basis to a collection that will, in subsequent chapters, examine not just the practice but also the abstract implications of breath that arise in more philosophical discourse.

Laying the foundation for this eclectic dialogue is the straightforward account of the anatomical reality of breath function by Dr Yolanda Heman-Ackah. From the vantage point of her position as a practising otolaryngologist (ear, nose and throat specialist), she provides a base line of information from which all healthy breathing practice can develop. In her illustrated chapter she examines the medical science background to the breath, with a particular focus on its implications for the laryngeal structures involved in vocal production. In so doing, she signals not only the importance of breath in preventative care but also in relation to ensuring the optimal performance of the vocal mechanism, a factor sometimes missed by those involved solely with the malfunctioning end of the health spectrum.

Dr Hemen-Ackah takes a position about the muscles of breath support, particularly the transversus abdominis, with which other practitioners have subsequently been able to take issue as a result of evidence that has recently come to light provided by new observational opportunities, such as electromyographic and ultrasound measuring. Up-to-the-minute research about this group of muscles has revealed that the most important muscle in terms of passive support and active expiration is the transversus abdominis. Dudley Knight of the University of California at Irvine, usefully indicates in a discussion with the editors the newly discovered fact that, far from being for torso stabilization only, with the internal and external obliques as primary abdominal muscles of expiration, the transversus should now be regarded as being the primary muscle of expiration. Professor Knight, thereby, draws crucial attention to the importance of a dialogue between the work of the scientists and those practising in the creative and therapeutic arts in order that both sides can benefit from the discoveries and experiences of the other.

Dr John Costello, a physician in respiratory sciences at King's College, London, confirmed a need for this exchange of information between the arts and sciences in his key-note address at the Performance Breath Conference at the Royal Academy of Dramatic Art on 5 January 2007. In his speech, he particularly noted the scarcity of a meaningful dialogue between the medical sciences and those voice practitioners situated in the humanities. He drew attention to the medical scientist who looks at breath solely as pathology, i.e. airway disease, lung diseases and cancer and the voice trainer who views breath in a holistic context as a healthful means of both voicing and 'being'. He made clear recommendations that this dichotomy should be investigated.

Many voice and holistic practitioners trainers, by way of a contrast to the medical sciences, have taken a wider look at the breath and drawn from many sources, including the neurosciences, respiratory sciences, the science of emotions, muscular-skeletal influences, functional physiology, acoustic studies, computer science, linguistics and so on. Whilst clearly this eclecticism can be fruitful, it also poses dilemmas about how to translate this knowledge into authoritative practice.

The challenge faced by all those involved with training has been one of translating such knowledge appropriately and ensuring that 'factual' information is sensitively communicated. In the light of growing knowledge about the brain that reveals the ways in which factual information is received in one part of the brain and not the other, where vocal and physical habits are processed, it becomes increasingly important to initiate sophisticated processes that will enable real and lasting change to actually take place based on more holistic approaches.

In this context, therefore, a conscious dialogue between the mind and the body (both utilizing the evidences of science and the experiences of the body) is advocated in order to help understand existing patterns of vocal and physical connection and to help create new ones. This approach mirrors those taken elsewhere in holistic practice where subjective experiences are set alongside scientific evidences and their practical applications in order to provide a fuller picture. It also demonstrates the importance of distinguishing between the strands of the field of breath studies outlined in the following chapters so that their role within a collective synthesis of thought can be clearly seen (Siegel 2007, p. xvi).

Dr Stephanie Martin's chapter adds to this body of thought from a speech and language scientist's perspective with a cradle to the grave account that examines the place of breath in both the diagnostic process and the remedial process in relation to the voice within speech and language sciences. By bridging various disciplines, this chapter clearly supports the idea of making the invisible breath visible in an exploration of its contribution to voice from a mechanical, 'cause and effect' perspective. Dr Martin is also, however, keenly aware that by highlighting just one aspect of an integrated system, such as voice, it should not dilute the contribution of other factors that affect breath capacity, support and control examined in greater detail elsewhere in the book.

Following on are two chapters from the perspective of the Alexander Technique by April Pierrot and Jessica Wolf respectively, offering both anatomical illustration and evidence of practice where the work on the breath in the context of the technique reveals obvious differences to clients' physical and mental health. The clear relationship between a health giving application of the breath and the enhancement of performance for both the actor and the lawyer in the case studies offered, demonstrates the enduring effectiveness of the Alexander Technique in a preventative health care role wherever breath is consciously applied.

BIBLIOGRAPHY

Siegel, Daniel J. (2007) *The Mindful Brain*. Preface. New York: WW Norton and Company

CHAPTER 1

The Science of Breath and the Voice

YOLANDA D. HEMAN-ACKA

WITH ILLUSTRATIONS BY TROY OHLSON

INTRODUCTION

My interest in breath and the professional voice began with my own voice difficulties and with increasing awareness of the vocal difficulties of many of my friends. I have a mild paresis (nerve weakness) of one of my vocal folds, which made it extremely difficult for me to project my voice, access my breath for support and vary the pitch of my voice. This weakness in my vocal fold affected my ability to communicate effectively, leaving many new acquaintances with a first impression of me as a meek, quiet individual who is unsure of herself. The limited vocal inflection would occasionally leave those who knew me well with the impression that I was angry or uninterested in conversation. Each of these impressions was far from the truth and it was very difficult for me to correct these deficiencies in my voice, despite my active efforts to do so.

Unfortunately, most of general otolaryngology (ear, nose and throat care) that is taught and practised around the world today does not address voice care and many otolaryngologists (ear, nose and throat doctors) are unaware of how to diagnose and treat subtle voice problems, particularly those that affect individuals who rely on their voice for their profession. Like many voice professionals, I sought care from my otolaryngology colleagues and came up with no answers. It was then that my quest for knowledge began. After I completed my residency in otolaryngology, I did an extra year of fellowship training in professional voice care with Robert T. Sataloff, M.D., D.M.A. As part of my training, I participated in singing voice therapy, singing voice lessons, speaking voice therapy and acting voice lessons. I was examined by Dr Sataloff and was diagnosed with vocal fold paresis, a diagnosis that at least three very prominent and well-respected otolaryngologists had missed previously. It was this weakness in my vocal folds that was limiting my ability to speak loudly without sounding like I was yelling, limiting my ability to talk for long periods of time without feeling as though I was running out of breath or straining my voice and limiting my ability to vary the inflection in my voice that would allow me to accurately express my emotions and personality through my voice. Despite progress with voice therapy, I needed voice surgery to help support my weak vocal fold and restore my ability to project my voice and vary its pitch. What I learned from this experience is that professional voice users need to be educated about both normal, healthy voice production and abnormal, disordered voice production and the medical conditions that can affect them both. I define a 'voice professional' as anyone who relies on their voice to carry out the day-to-day functions of their profession. These may include teachers, lawyers, telemarketers, stock brokers, investors, physicians, judges, actors, singers, salespersons and politicians. It is important not only to have this knowledge base, but also to know how to apply it in everyday practice. This chapter describes how the breath, the larynx, the body and the basic principles of sound production interact to produce the voice.

THE MECHANICS OF VOICE PRODUCTION

In my practice, I focus on breath as it assists the voice user in producing the most healthy and efficient sound. In may be helpful then to look first at the mechanics of sound and work our way back to the significant impact of the breath.

The production of voice involves a similar set of mechanics as the production of sound from any source. Let's look at a couple of musical instruments, for example, the trumpet and the clarinet. Each instrument has a power source that serves to produce airflow. In both cases this is the flow of air from the musician's mouth. Each instrument also has a sound source or oscillator that moves the stream of air into a sound wave, which is a rhythmic movement of air through space. Each sound wave has a height (or amplitude) that goes from high to low rhythmically and repeatedly in a predictable rate of recurrence (the frequency). In the example of musical instruments, the reed in the clarinet and the two lips buzzing together in the mouthpiece of a trumpet serve the purpose of being an oscillator. Finally each instrument has a resonating chamber through which the sound waves travel. As the sound waves travel through the resonance chamber, they bounce back and forth off its walls. The result is that some of the sound waves get bigger amplitudes as they bounce back and forth and other sound waves become dampened by this process. By augmenting some sound waves and dampening others, the resonating chamber shapes the final quality of the sound that is produced, resulting in a sound that is unique to the instrument producing it. Thus, the shape of the clarinet produces sounds that allow one to differentiate that sound as being distinctively different from the sound produced by the shape of the trumpet. At the end of the sound source is the amplifier. The amplifier is usually shaped like a megaphone. As the sound waves leave the sound source, they bounce back and forth against the walls of the amplifier, which causes them to gain height. This greater height (or amplitude) is interpreted by the human ear as being a louder sound. In the case of the trumpet and the clarinet, the bell at the end of the instrument is the amplifier.

In voice production, the source of airflow is provided primarily by the lungs. The abdominal muscles, chest and back help to generate the force necessary to produce an adequate and controlled flow of air for voice production. Like the buzzing lips in the mouthpiece of the trumpet, the sound source or oscillator is the vocal folds, which sit inside the voice box and move rhythmically and place the air from the lungs into a wave-like motion. The resonance chamber and amplifier are produced by the remainder of the vocal tract: the supraglottis (the space in the voice box above the vocal folds); the pharynx or throat; the oral cavity including the tongue and palate, the nasal cavity, the sinuses and the head.

THE BREATH AS A SOURCE OF AIRFLOW

Once we have an understanding of the mechanics of sound, we can more clearly appreciate the supremacy of breath in both vocal communication and in holistic practice. An exhaled breath is the airflow that provides the power for voice production. Breathing involves a complex interplay between the lungs, the abdomen, the chest, the back, the legs and hips, as well as other structures. A look at the specifics of each system will allow us to understand how their delicate interplay is the basis for all vocal sound production.

THE LUNGS

The lungs (see Figure 1.1) have the ability to expand in all three dimensions: upward/downward, sideways and forward/backward. The greatest area for excursion of the lungs is down. The lungs are housed within the chest, are separated from the abdomen (the belly) by a muscle called the diaphragm and are encased on all sides by the ribs. Because the ribs are bony and do not stretch easily, they limit the amount of outward expansion of the lungs, leaving the greatest room for expansion down, into the abdomen. The abdomen is a cavity that holds the stomach, liver, bladder and intestines. Because all of the walls of the abdomen are made of muscle, there is a lot of room for stretch and expansion inside of the abdominal cavity. The diaphragm moves down with inhalation (taking a breath in) and moves up with exhalation (letting a breath out). As the diaphragm moves down with inhalation, the abdominal contents are pushed downward

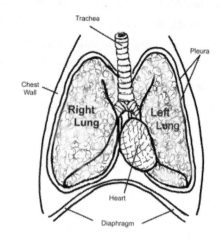

Figure 1.1

and outward to allow room for the expanding lungs. The movement of the diaphragm downward increases the negative pressure in the chest, creating a suction effect in the chest. As the diaphragm moves down into the abdomen, the abdominal muscles relax and stretch outward and more air is siphoned into the lungs as the person breathes in. During normal breathing, exhalation is passive. That is, the diaphragm simply relaxes, causing it to come back up into the chest, which causes a release of air from the lungs. This action is similar to the way in which releasing the fingers holding closed the opening of a balloon will allow for the passive flow of air out of the balloon, without any need for external force or pushing on the side walls of the balloon. With active exhalation, such as is used with the 'supported breath' commonly used by singers and actors to help project the voice, abdominal force is used to assist with pushing air out of the lungs. Using the balloon analogy again, this would be similar to squeezing the sides of the balloon as the fingers are released at the open end of the balloon to force the air out in a faster and more voluminous stream. Larger and consciously controlled breaths use muscles in both the diaphragm and abdomen. Every day, shallow breaths use diaphragmatic breathing almost exclusively. In voice production, a greater control of airflow and, thus, the voice, can be achieved with abdominal breathing patterns than with passive breathing alone.

The abdominal region provides the greatest room for expansion of the lungs. The lungs consist of two halves, the right and the left. The right lung is divided further into three lobes, while the left lung is divided into two lobes only. Each lobe functions much like a balloon, expanding when air enters during inhalation and shrinking when air leaves during exhalation. Like balloons, the lobes of the lung have a certain degree of elasticity, which allows this expansion and recoil. The lower lobes of the lungs have the greatest capacity for volume and also have the greatest ability to expand (the compliance). For instance, two balloons with the same volume capacity but with different thickness of the balloon wall will differ in the amount of energy and force it takes to blow up the balloons. It will be harder to blow up the thicker walled balloon (which has less compliance) and easier to blow-up the thinner walled balloon (which has greater compliance). Thus, the same force of air will put more air volume into the thinner walled balloon (high compliance) than it will into the thicker walled (low compliance) balloon. The higher compliance of the lower lobes of the lung allows for greater expansion into the abdomen. The ribs surround the top lobes of the lungs, thus, limiting their ability to expand and recoil upward and outward. The positioning of the collarbones and the scapulae (the shoulder blades) also limits the expansion of the lungs backward. The optimal position for maximal expansion of the lungs during deep breathing is with both the collarbones and the scapulae flat, down and maximally expanded horizontally, to allow for maximal pulmonary expansion and filling.

In addition to the alignment issue note above, lung function can be limited further by physical pathologies such as asthma and chronic obstructive pulmonary disease (which results from smoking). In such cases, the elasticity of the lungs is limited, but the capacity remains the same. Thus, the lungs are able to inhale the same amount of air; however, the force produced on exhalation is decreased due to limited recoil within the lungs. Restrictive lung diseases, such as emphysema (a longer-term sequela of smoking), obesity and the effects of broken ribs, limit the amount of air the lungs can inhale and thus, the amount of air the lungs can exhale. Each of these then affects airflow and control during voice production and impairments can predispose to a soft voice, vocal fatigue and decreased vocal projection.

THE ABDOMEN

Another major component of the integrated breath system is the abdomen (see Figure 1.2). The abdomen contributes to breathing by helping to control the flow of air on exhalation, which is the point in the breathing cycle when speaking occurs. The abdomen consists of several layers of muscles: the external oblique, the internal oblique, the transverse abdominus and the rectus abdominus muscles. The external oblique muscles lie immediately beneath the

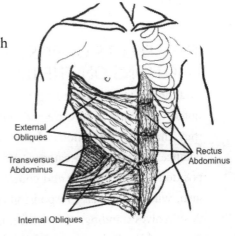

Figure 1.2

skin and fat. The internal oblique muscles lie beneath the external obliques and run horizontally along the side of the abdomen. Much of the abdominal contribution to breathing is from the internal and external obliques. The rectus abdominus muscles lie in the centre of the abdomen with their fibers running vertically from the pubic bone to the breast bone (sternum). The rectus abdominus muscle bends the body forward and is the main muscle used during sit-ups. Its main function is to support the back and to assist with balance; it does not appear to contribute much to breathing. Under the internal oblique muscles lie the transverse abdominal muscles, which contribute mostly to core strengthening. Sustained contraction of the abdomen during exhalation helps to regulate the flow of air from the lungs during breathing and phonation.

Another important side note for the voice user is that knowledge of the abdominal anatomy and musculature is critical for the voice professional who is considering abdominal surgery. Surgery on the abdomen weakens the muscles that are cut. Rehabilitation and strengthening of the weakened abdominal muscles prior to resuming a normal vocal routine is imperative to helping to maintain vocal health and to preventing vocal fold injury after abdominal surgery, especially for professional voice users.

THE BACK

The next major component of the integrated breath system is the back, which consists of five to six layers of muscles whose fibers cross each other. The main function of the back is to help maintain balance and to serve as a support for the abdomen. Abdominal support of breathing requires the support of the back muscles to maximize the force of any given abdominal contractile effort. If firm support from the back occurs simultaneously with pressure from the abdomen, a greater force is created.

THE EFFECTS OF POSTURE, BALANCE, STANCE AND EMOTIONS ON THE BREATH AND THE VOICE

In addition to understanding the key components of the breath system, it must be noted that shifts in posture and stance affect the position of one's centre of gravity, thus changing the actions of the muscles that are engaged actively in maintaining balance. For optimal breathing and voice production, posture and stance should be positioned to limit sway and contraction of the torso muscles of the back and abdomen, with the primary responsibility for balance falling on the leg muscles. Ideally, this involves standing with the feet flat on the floor with the weight forward over the metatarsal heads (balls of the feet), shoulder width apart, knees slightly bent and torso erect and lifted. This results in a stable stance with the centre of gravity residing at about the centre of the pelvis. Standing with the feet together and knees straight shifts the centre of gravity upwards and the back and abdominal muscles become more actively involved in maintaining balance, thus limiting stability and support for voice production (see Figure 1.3). Keeping the centre of gravity low frees the back and abdominal muscles to be used more effectively. In doing so, this allows the abdomen and back muscles to be used primarily for breathing and breath support and less so for maintaining balance. This is the principle behind many of the different acting, singing and dance techniques and exercises for posture and breathing.

Dizziness and/or imbalance that are caused by medications, alcohol, drugs, neuropathies, inner ear disease and/or visual dysfunction can cause excessive engagement of the back and abdominal muscles as the body attempts to maintain its balance, thus lessening the use of these muscles for breath support. Anxiety, fear, grief and other emotions involve tension in many of the muscles in the back and the abdomen and also alter the breathing pattern. This alteration in the breathing pattern can affect the ability to control the voice, resulting in a soft, quavering, or poorly projected voice.

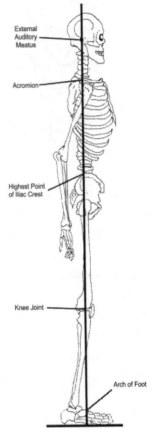

External Auditory Meatus

Acromion

Highest Point of Iliac Crest

Knee Joint

Arch of Foot

Figure 1.3

THE SOUND SOURCE: THE OSCILLATOR

Similar to the trumpet, which needs the buzzing lips to serve as the oscillator for sound production, the human voice has the vocal folds to serve this function. The larynx, which is commonly called the voice box, houses the vocal folds and is the primary organ involved in voice production. It is encased by the 'Adam's apple' (also called the thyroid cartilage) and sits above the trachea (the windpipe) and in front of the esophagus (the swallowing tube) in the neck (see Figure 1.4).

The movements of the vocal folds themselves are coordinated by the activities of the cartilages, the muscles and the nerves of the larynx. The hyoid bone is the only free floating bone in the body, not articulating with any other bone, only with

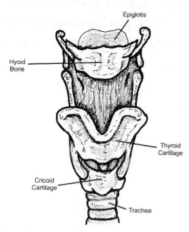

Figure 1.4

muscles, which themselves are attached to other bones and cartilages. Muscles from the hyoid (the digastric and strap muscles, respectively), connect the larynx to the skull base and jaw above and to the clavicle and scapulae below. The hyoid has the capacity to move up and down as the muscles that connect to it contract, but it does not participate directly in movement of the vocal folds.

Three cartilages provide the structural support for the muscles and mucus membranes of the larynx similar to the way in which the framework of the house provides support for the walls and floors. The main cartilages of the larynx are the thyroid, cricoid and arytenoids. The two pyramid-shaped arytenoid cartilages sit on top of the cricoid and serve as points of attachment for most of the muscles that are involved in voice production. The laryngeal muscles move the arytenoid cartilages and this results in opening and closing of the vocal folds. The cricoid provides the base of support of the larynx. The cricoid sits on top of the trachea and is shaped like a signet ring, being larger in the back than it is in the front. The cricoid is a stable structure in the neck. The thyroid cartilage can be made to rock upon it as pitch is varied.

The thyroid, the largest of the cartilages, is shield-shaped and is open in the back. The thyroid cartilage is the anatomical 'voice box' that houses and serves as protection for the vocal folds. This cartilage is very prominent in men and is also commonly called the Adam's apple. The vocal folds themselves attach inside the voice box to the thyroid cartilage in front and to the arytenoid cartilages in back.

There are muscles inside the larynx (the intrinsic muscles) and some outside the larynx (the extrinsic muscles) that manage the complex movements of the larynx. The extrinsic strap muscles raise and lower the larynx to help with swallowing. These muscles also are used with excessive yelling or screaming and other sounds produced by straining the voice. The intrinsic muscles move the vocal folds to open, close, lengthen and tense them during voice production.

Actual phonation, the creation of sound, requires a complex interaction between the larynx and many other bodily systems to achieve the sound that we associate with the voice. This physical integration is an aspect of vocal production that many professional voice users do not fully grasp. The sound of the voice is produced by the movement of the vocal folds in the larynx as air is forced past them from the lungs.

THE OSCILLATING VOCAL FOLDS

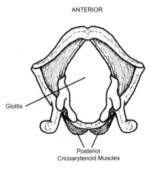

ANTERIOR

Glottis

Posterior
Cricoarytenoid Muscles

Vocal Folds Open

Figure 1.5

The sound source for voice production is the vocal folds. Though this fact is relatively straightforward, the structure of the vocal folds themselves is less commonly known. Knowledge of structure of the folds provides an understanding, which can lead to more accurate and specific care and use of the voice. The vocal folds sit inside the thyroid cartilage and span from the front of the thyroid cartilage, to the back of the larynx, where they attach to the arytenoid cartilages. The rate at which the vocal folds vibrate determines the pitch of the voice. A greater number of vibrations per second results in a higher vocal pitch. Conversely, a lesser number of vibrations of the vocal folds per second corresponds to a lower vocal pitch.

Previously, the vocal folds were called 'vocal cords'. However, the term 'vocal cord' is somewhat outdated and not commonly used by medical professionals today because it is not an accurate description of their function. Instead of vibrating like the cords of a violin string or piano, the vocal folds actually move more in a wavelike motion, similar to the movement of buzzing lips. It is the movement of vocal folds in a wavelike motion over the underlying vocal ligament that is responsible for the production of sound in the larynx. During breathing (see Figure 1.5), the vocal folds are open, meaning that there is a space between them to allow air to pass into the lungs for breathing. During phonation, the two edges of the vocal folds come together and are approximated, eliminating the space between them and allowing only a small stream of air to pass each time the vocal folds vibrate (see Figure 1.6). As the sound travels through the remainder of the vocal tract (the throat and mouth), it resonates and certain frequencies are amplified, giving the voice its character. This produces the sound that we associate with the voice and that gives each person his or her own characteristic voice that allows one to identify the individual based on the sound of the voice alone.

How the breath is manipulated is a key factor in determining the relative loudness of the voice. A louder voice can be produced by one of two methods: by increasing the airflow from the lungs or by increasing the force of closure of the vocal folds. The preferred method of increasing the volume of the voice utilizes a combination of both strategies, with a primary focus on increasing airflow. A greater force in the air stream from the lungs causes the vocal folds to oscillate back and forth more widely as they vibrate, resulting in a louder voice. When less airflow is used from the lungs, the vocal folds oscillate during vibration to a lesser degree and a softer sound is produced.

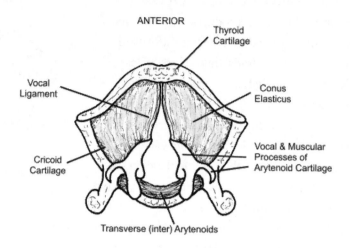

ANTERIOR

Thyroid
Cartilage

Vocal
Ligament

Conus
Elasticus

Cricoid
Cartilage

Vocal & Muscular
Processes of
Arytenoid Cartilage

Transverse (inter) Arytenoids

Vocal Folds Closed

Figure I.6

The other way to increase volume is to increase the force of closure of the vocal folds. However, doing so is dangerous to the vocal folds and places one at risk for developing tears, bleeding, nodules, scars and other lesions on the vocal folds. Oftentimes, forceful closing of the vocal folds involves using other muscles in the throat and neck, in addition to the laryngeal muscles, to produce the voice. These muscles may include those in the throat, neck, tongue and the larynx itself. Such use of excess force is termed supraglottic hyperfunction (and also is referred to commonly as muscle tension dysphonia) and strains the vocal folds. Consequently, the professional voice user should learn how to use the voice efficiently by taking voice lessons, acting classes and/or voice therapy to obtain an optimal balance between airflow forces and the force of vocal fold closure to preserve vocal health.

If the vocal folds do not close completely when they vibrate, as can be caused by a mild vocal fold weakness (paresis), vocal fold masses (such as a polyp, nodule, or cyst), vocal fold scar, or vocal fold swelling, then there may be escape of air as the vocal folds vibrate. In such instances, a greater degree of airflow is required from the lungs to produce the same volume of voice. Thus, the same degree of effort from the lungs produces a softer sounding voice. Many people who have incomplete closure of the vocal folds during phonation experience vocal fatigue with prolonged voice use, decreased ability to project the voice and decreased ability to use effective breath support.

The behaviour of the vocal folds during phonation can be understood through a stepped process of visualization. First, the airflow used for voice production can be imagined as behaving like the stream of water that comes out of the end of a water hose. Second, by imagining that there is a hole in the water hose, it can be seen that the water emerging out of the end of the hose will have a weaker stream and a more shallow projection area because of water lost elsewhere in the system. In order to produce the same volume of water stream and the same area of projection of the water as occurs with an unbroken hose, more water will clearly need to be pumped through to compensate for the water that will be lost. From a voice perspective, this image helps us to understand that a greater requirement for increased airflow from the lungs is instigated when a gap exists between the vocal folds. When the vocal folds are perfectly symmetric and meet in the midline there is no gap but when there is, there is a loss of airflow. From a functional perspective, incomplete vocal fold closure means that more energy is needed to produce greater airflow from the lungs to increase volume and projection and to sustain phonation, which creates a greater susceptibility to fatigue. Many people with incomplete glottic closure subconsciously compensate by using muscles in the neck, throat and tongue to produce a louder voice and then begin to suffer the consequences of laryngeal hyperfunction, as well as those associated with incomplete closure. This pattern leads to voice fatigue, vocal strain, chronic hoarseness and sometimes to serious vocal fold injury.

THE VOCAL TRACT AS RESONATOR AND AMPLIFIER

To follow our musical instrument analogy to the final component, the human equivalent of the trumpet horn and bell is the vocal tract, which acts as both the resonance chamber and the amplifier. The vocal tract includes the pharynx (throat), tongue, palate (roof of the mouth), mouth, nose, and to a lesser degree, the sinuses and the head. As sound waves travel through the vocal tract from the larynx, they bounce back and forth along the walls of the vocal tract. As the sound resonates throughout the vocal tract, it gains energy in those areas that are amplified by the particular shape of the vocal tract and loses energy in those areas that are dampened by the shape of the vocal tract. Because everyone's throat, mouth, nose and head are shaped differently, resonance of the voice occurs at different sites in the vocal tract and to different degrees from one person to another. This resonance is responsible for giving each voice its own 'signature' sound that allows us to distinguish one individual from another and its 'ring', which allows the voice to be heard even in the presence of a significant degree of background noise, such as a singer singing above an orchestra or an actor performing live in an open theatre.

Amplification of the voice occurs primarily in the mouth, which has a megaphone-like effect on vocal projection. In general, a more open mouth causes greater amplification of the voice. This is achieved best by optimizing the position of the tongue, the palate, the jaw and the lips so that the tongue sits forward and flat, the palate is elevated, the jaw is maximally open, and the lips are relaxed yet open. Elongation and widening of the vocal tract includes several conscious mechanisms, including maintaining correct neck posture. If the neck is tilted back or the chin is lifted too high, a bend is created in the throat, which effectively narrows the resonance and amplifying chamber at the region of the tongue base. Ideally, the head should be in the neutral position, straight up and down, so that the spine is straight through the skull base. This produces a straighter vocal tract and usually enhances resonance and projection. Elevation of the palate helps to open the vocal tract in the back of the mouth and seals the nasal cavity to minimize a nasal-sounding voice. Relaxation of the tongue base, with the tip of the tongue placed in a more forward (but relaxed) position, helps to lengthen the back of the mouth and widen the space at the tongue base, creating a longer, greater diameter amplifier.

SUMMARY

The voice is produced by a complex interplay between the breath, the vocal folds and the vocal tract. Many organ systems in the body participate actively in voice production in addition to the larynx, and each has a vital role. Acquiring knowledge of how the voice is produced and its relationship to the breath is the first step in understanding how to care for and maintain the voice throughout one's life. The voice is the means by which humans express their emotions and communicate with each other. The breath is the means by which the voice is able to convey these sentiments. Thus, the breath, the voice and emotion are all intimately related and reliant upon each other.

BIBLIOGRAPHY

Gould, W.J. and Okamura, H. (1973) 'Static Lung Volumes in Singers' *Annals of Otology, Rhinology and Laryngology 82*(1): 89–95.

Hirano, M. (1997) 'Structure and Vibratory Pattern of the Vocal Folds.' In N. Sawashima and F.S. Cooper (eds) *Dynamic Aspects of Speech Production*. Tokyo: University of Tokyo Press.

Hixon, T.J. and Hoffman, C. (1978) 'Chest Wall Shape During Singing.' In V. Lawrence (ed.) *Transcripts of the Seventh Annual Symposium, Care of the Professional Voice*. New York: The Voice Foundation.

Sataloff, R.T. (1997) *Professional Voice: The Science and Art of Clinical Care*, Second Edition. San Diego: Singular Publishing Group, Inc.

Sundberg, J. (1977) 'The Acoustics of the Singing Voice.' *Scientific American 236*.

Sundberg, J. (1997) 'Vocal Tract Resonance.' In R.T. Sataloff (ed.) *Professional Voice: The Science and Art of Clinical Care*, 2nd edn. San Diego: Singular Publishing Group, Inc.

West, J.B. (1985) 'Mechanics of Breathing.' In J.B. West (ed.) *Best and Taylor's Physiological Basis of Medical Practice*, 11th edn. Baltimore: Williams and Wilkins.

CHAPTER 2

A Short History of Breath from Womb to Tomb

STEPHANIE MARTIN

The focus of this chapter is predominately to look at the way in which breath underpins voice. By exploring how the role and constituents of this vocal 'scaffold' change throughout life, it is hoped to offer an overarching perspective, which will be of interest to those whose practice recognizes the importance of the voice in determining the physical, mental and psychological health of those with whom they work. These may be practitioners from the world of alternative and holistic health and from the more circumscribed world of voice, either artistic or clinical.

Each one of us has a voice that is unique, one that can be instantly identified as belonging to us by those whom we know. At times, when an individual is unknown to us, we create a picture of them from hearing their voice. In Shakespeare's *A Midsummer Night's Dream*, Pyramus says, ' I see a voice': and indeed on hearing a voice we often may 'see' an individual. Sometimes that picture is inaccurate and the tall and dark individual turns out to be small and fair skinned but the voice has the ability to engage our senses of hearing, vision and emotion in a particularly 'immediate' way. We can affect vocal quality and voice use by altering pitch, resonance, volume, intonation, speed and pace while still retaining the voice and communication style which identify it as our own. Our voice serves to reflect not only our emotional state, our personality and our physical state, but also our previous life history and experience. Voice is a critical indicator of both physiological and psychological well-being and as such offers a particularly acute and effective gauge of physical and mental health. This point is usefully summarized by Mathieson (2001, p. 4), 'In adulthood the voice eventually provides an amalgam of personal information'.

Voice production is dependent on three different systems, respiratory, phonatory and resonatory, working together in order to communicate effectively. The integrated nature of voice production is of particular importance to those working with the damaged voice. All contributory factors within an individual's environment (here the term environment is used in its widest sense to encompass the individual's vocal, social, physical and psychological environment), need to be evaluated in order to determine the possible impact of each in terms of its collective contribution to, or maintenance of a voice disorder. A vocal problem is rarely the result of a single specific factor; therefore to limit intervention to one element of an integrated system would be counter-productive.

Breathing for speech and singing are of course modifications of the main purpose of the respiratory system, which is to maintain life by the metabolic exchange of the gases, oxygen and carbon dioxide. The balance of oxygen and carbon dioxide is constantly changing with bodily activity and this balance is adjusted by the central nervous system. The primary function of the larynx is to protect the airway and maintain life and this may be seen in the number and complexity of the protective laryngeal reflex mechanisms that exist. This protective 'valving' by the vocal folds is achieved through the action of the intrinsic and extrinsic laryngeal muscles. The resistance that varying degrees of valving provide affects breathing patterns and this in turn affects voice production. On occasion this protective valving action can lead to voice disorders, for example, excessive coughing can result in trauma to the vocal folds, causing swelling and oedema, which in turn will interfere with the normal vibratory pattern of the vocal folds. In certain neurological conditions, random rapid movements of the vocal folds at rest may 'interrupt' normal respiration, which may threaten life and will certainly interfere with the vibratory patterns of the vocal folds and thus affect phonation.

This chapter will explore this symbiosis of breath and voice. It will examine the direct or indirect effect of breath capacity, support and control on vocal quality as a result of psychological, physiological and environmental demands. As Hixon (1987) suggests, within the broad spectrum of physiological function in speech, respiration is involved in the regulation of parameters such as intensity, fundamental frequency, linguistic stress and the division of speech into various units. All these features are important diagnostic 'markers'. Breath may therefore be both a sign and a symptom of a voice disorder. Colton and Casper (1996) include the term 'breathy' in a list of nine major primary symptoms of voice problems, along with hoarseness, reduced phonational range, aphonia, pitch breaks or inappropriately high pitch, strain/struggle voice, tremor, pain and other physical symptoms. The authors also include 'breathy' or 'breathiness' in an overarching list of perceptual signs, that is signs that are judged by the listener as a characteristic of an individual's voice. The other signs they propose are pitch, loudness, quality, other behaviours and aphonia. For the clinician, inefficient breath capacity, control and support can suggest a vocal pathology so the assessment of breathing patterns, breath capacity, breath control and breath support is a critical measure not only in terms of diagnosis, but also in terms of therapy outcome.

Breath may thus be referenced in terms of its role in initiating and sustaining voice and its role as a measure of vocal quality. This dual role is of considerable diagnostic importance for the clinician but it must always be seen within the context of an overall profile of a client's vocal health, a profile gained from perceptual, acoustic and physiological investigation, in addition to the client's own history of the voice problem.

Our life source is our breath, the breath that gives us voice, yet the breath of those that gave us life also gave us our voice. Our DNA determines our physiological inheritance, which dictates the size and shape of the vocal tract. The anatomical features of the vocal tract in turn determine the individual's unique vocal 'fingerprint', the vocal quality that distinguishes one individual from another and which cannot be completely suppressed or disguised. Other inherited physiological factors that might affect the vocal tract are congenital disorders such as cranio-facial abnormalities, palatal abnormalities such as cleft palate or sub-mucous cleft, laryngeal abnormalities such as, laryngeal webs or asymmetry of the larynx, syndromes such as Down's or tracheal abnormalities such as tracheo-oesophageal fistula or stenosis. It is also important to consider the influence of pre-disposing factors on voice quality. These are factors that are not, as have been described above, implicated in altered vocal quality due to the configuration of the vocal tract, but are those that indirectly affect voice quality for example poor respiratory competence, allergic conditions such as asthma or enlarged adenoids.

How we hear or respond to sound and our ability to interpret sound is important in determining how we perceive, monitor, modify and use our voice. While our inherited vocal tract configuration will not allow significant voice quality change, limited voice quality change is possible through muscular adjustment of the vocal tract. Our inherited ability to interpret sound allows certain individuals to adjust vocal parameters such as pitch, volume and intonation with innate skill, for others this process must be learned. The 'elite' vocal performer (Koufman 1998) has an innate vocal ability not only to produce a wonderful sound but their proprioceptive and kinaesthetic inheritance allows them to perceive, monitor and modify this sound. For others, due, for example, to a congenital disorder such as deafness, their ability to access this rich inheritance will be compromised.

The voice we inherit is, therefore, predetermined by our DNA, and is also the result of personality characteristics, emotional reactions to acute or chronic life stressors and emotional disturbances. The voice we acquire, however, is shaped by our communicative competence – our ability, desire or need to communicate. All of these aspects of our voice, whether inherited or acquired, affect the movement of the vocal folds through increased levels of intrinsic and extrinsic laryngeal muscle tension. As a consequence of these changing tension levels, a spiral of change occurs in patterns of respiration, which in turn bring about change in vocal patterns.

No dynamic structure is impervious to the influence of internal and external forces and so it is with the voice. Voice, from infancy to senescence, is affected by anatomical and physiological changes. These changes are a consequence of a number of factors, which include the ageing process, disease and disorder. Breath and breathing determine physical as well as vocal health, for example, lack of efficient oxygenation of the blood due to respiratory inefficiency reduces the biomechanical efficiency of the body. Breath is a pivotal force in phonation, part of the mechanical 'cause and effect' which contributes to changes in vocal quality and communicative competence. It is important to remember that changes in voice quality are affected from infancy to old age by changes related to a number of different factors including general health, vocal health, vocal history, vocal care, vocal demand, vocal status (the individual's perception of their voice), voice geneogram (family and cultural values), social functioning, anxiety and stress and the environment (Martin and Lockhart 2005).

The integrated nature of breath and phonation means that as voice and phonation change, so too does respiration. The following section beginning with the infant voice, offers a brief overview of the link between breath and voice as a consequence of growth, health, lifestyle, ageing, disease and illness through infancy, adolescence, adulthood and old age.

The infant voice is controlled through crying. The infant larynx positioned high in the vocal tract is a pliable structure with short vocal folds (which determines the high pitch of the infant voice) and limited neuromuscular coordination. This results in limited control over the tension of the vocal folds and the air pressure required for speech, resulting in short bursts of often quite loud sound. Despite its limited repertoire, the infant 'voice' can accurately reflect respiratory, neurological and maturational status. Since the lungs are the last major organs to mature in the womb, breathing complications are common during the first few hours and days of a premature baby's life. Through improving gas exchange in the lungs and increasing the level of oxygen delivery treatment options in very premature infants (through mechanical ventilation/intubation of the lungs) are usually successful. Due however, to the fragility of the infant's lungs, intubation may sometimes cause complications which can result in permanent damage to the lungs; chronic neonatal lung disease may result in oxygen dependency for many years. This extended period of intubation can in turn cause scarring and changes in the tissue of the vocal tract leading to hoarseness. Respiratory instability, respiratory tract problems and poor respiratory control, prompt concern and invite further examination, as they may indicate congenital anomalies of the vocal tract such as papillomas or laryngeal webs. Similarly impaired vocal fold movement, high-pitched cries (sometimes one or two octaves above that of a normal infant), unusual melodic patterns and unstable vocal signals should be investigated, as these may be symptoms of specific syndromes. One such syndrome, although rare is cri-du-chat, characterized, as the name suggests, by a high-pitched cry similar to that of a cat.

As the infant matures and vocalisations turn into babble, voice and speech problems may become apparent through rhythm, intonation and breath patterns which differ from the norm. Damage to the central nervous system, which has occurred before, during, or shortly after birth and which may result in cognitive and cerebral dysfunction, may present in voice and speech delays and disorders characterized by hypo-function of the laryngeal mechanism. Hypo-function is described by Andrews (1995, p. 168) as, 'inadequate muscular tone in the laryngeal mechanism and associated structures or systems'. In terms of respiration, there may be the use of an ingressive air stream for voicing, quick shallow inhalation, inefficient control of exhalation, or air may escape in a rush at the beginning of an utterance. These aberrant breathing patterns will result in an abrupt initiation of phonation, inappropriate or uncontrolled loudness and pitch, non-intentional pitch changes and the use of laryngeal valving, rather than respiratory muscle control of the exhaled air, leading to tension in the supraglottal resonators and an ensuing strident vocal quality. In sharp contrast, hyper-function of the laryngeal mechanism presents as 'a pervasive pattern of excessive effort and tension that affects many different structures and muscles' (Andrews 1995, p. 162). In the case of a hyper-functional breathing pattern, inhalation is limited with weak and short exhalation and reduced support and control of exhaled air. Increased muscular effort leads to voice problems; phonation is inconsistent with a breathy onset and excessive air escape, so the voice cuts in and out with limited audibility and minimal variation. There is often inadequate oral and nasal resonance and this lack of resonance may affect the intelligibility of speech sounds, as voiced and voiceless sounds are undifferentiated. In both, a lack of synchrony between respiration and the onset of phonation occurs.

Childhood disorders of resonance or of vocal quality, associated with reduced breath capacity and control, may also be the result of allergic conditions such as asthma. As a result of bronchial spasm, inflammation and oedema, respiration is compromised, leading to a reduction in airflow and vital capacity (VC). Vital capacity refers to the greatest amount of air that can be expelled from the lungs and airways after a maximum inspiration. This reduction in airflow and vital capacity in turn leads to reduced subglottic airflow leading to hyperfunctional phonation. Added to the effect on respiration, inflammation and oedema lead to increased vocal fold mass, which in turn affects voice quality. Asthma is not only a disorder of childhood – late onset asthma is an increasing feature of older age and the effect on respiration and voice is the same. While it is important to medicate to reduce breathing problems, the use of inhaled cortico-steroids particularly if delivered without the use of a spacer and without rinsing the mouth with water after use may result in alteration to vocal fold muscle tension (Harris 1992; Mathieson 2001). This additional respiratory loading is particularly important when seen within the context of the difference between children's and adults' speech breathing patterns. Mathieson (2001) notes that a four-year-old child exerts far more expiratory effort in speech breathing than adults and a child of seven uses relatively higher lung volumes to initiate vocal fold vibration than older children and adults.

Adolescent changes in vocal quality are the result of post-pubertal mutational changes, which occur in the female larynx due to the increased secretion of oestrogens and in the male larynx as a result of increased androgen secretion. An increase in the length of the vocal folds is noted particularly in the male, where the vocal folds can double in size. Changes in lung volume and vital capacity also occur – young adults have approximately four times the lung capacity of the five-year-old, while vital capacity is at its peak during the late teens and early twenties. Adolescent vocal quality and speech patterns are the result both of mutational and postural change. The very different picture of the open and proud posture of a six-year-old and that of an average 16-year-old is notable. Stereotypically adolescent body language is seen as an attempt either to withdraw by making themselves inconspicuous and occupying as little space as possible, or to assume a confidence they may not feel by taking up a greater amount of physical space. Both postures affect breath and therefore voice – lowered eye levels produce head/neck alignment changes that lead to a slumped spine and shallow breath, while the forward thrusting aggressive posture locks the neck and shoulders, affects respiration and limits easy onset of phonation. Youth culture is generally loud and vocally demanding. Alcohol, smoking and the effects from the use of recreational drugs such as cannabis or marijuana on the vocal folds will traumatize the upper respiratory track.

This cocktail of abusive vocal behaviour is not, of course, limited to adolescents; adults also energetically subscribe to this vocally traumatizing regime. Vocal challenges in adulthood may encompass muscular, neurological, skeletal, cardiovascular, respiratory and hormonal changes. All of which are reflected in the vocal tract and its supporting systems and vocal function.

For women, vocal change may be experienced as a result of changes in hormonal balance. During pregnancy, for example, voice quality change is temporary and is allied to the woman's reduced control and capacity over speech breathing due to the diaphragm's inability to descend on inspiration as pregnancy progresses. Postmenopausal permanent changes in voice quality occur due both to a reduction in female hormones and changes in the respiratory tract. Age-related changes are experienced by both men and women and are caused by a number of interrelated factors such as specific tissue structure changes within the vocal folds, changes within the lungs and a reduction in the mobility of the thoracic cage so the ribs become less mobile, leading to a breathy vocal quality. As always it must be remembered that age-related changes vary from individual to individual, so ageing does not have to equal vocal deterioration. It is not difficult to think of older professional voice users who have retained well-resonated voices, but it is worth noting that generally these individuals have retained good respiratory function.

Most major changes in vocal quality occur in the sixth and seventh decade as a result of muscular, skeletal and tissue changes, which result in reduced respiratory function and inevitably, affect the anatomy and physiology of phonation. As Mathieson notes, 'Respiratory disease can influence the speed and volume of inspiration and expiration so that both the sound of the voice and the timing of phonation are affected' (2001, p. 346)

By the age of 75 years respiratory efficiency is half that of a 30-year-old so there is less expendable air for phonation. Older people also experience increased reaction time and a decline in muscle strength so, as a result, changes occur in loudness, resonance, timing, pitch and vocal range. Vocal quality changes such as breathiness and roughness reflect incomplete closure of the glottis and loss of tension in the vocal folds.

'Breathy' vocal symptoms and perceptual signs may also be noted in a variety of acquired adult voice disorders such as chronic laryngitis, vocal nodules, vocal fold polyps, vocal fold cysts, vocal fold paresis, scarring of the vocal folds, laryngeal webs and bowing. Central nervous system dysfunction in conditions such as Parkinson's disease, or Multiple Sclerosis place many demands on respiration and the accompanying effect on voice is noted in altered loudness levels, changes in pace and pitch and loss of articulatory precision.

For those who work with 'damaged or disordered' voices, recognition of the importance of breath underpins both diagnostic and treatment options. When considering the aetiology of voice disorders, vocal symptoms are carefully assessed and respiratory function, in its widest sense, is a critical element of any diagnosis. Into this equation detailed information about a number of aspects of an individual's current and previous life style, voice use and response to external stress factors, needs to be factored. It is important to consider the impact of life circumstances on voice and voice on life circumstances and to this end it is often useful to produce a Voice Impact Profile (Martin and Lockhart 2005). Such a profile provides a subjective qualitative measure to build a more complete picture of a client, which may be used alongside data collected from other sources. Due to the visual representation of the results, specific areas of concern can be identified which will inform the clinical journey and validate change over time.

Breath offers a unique template for voice. Breath, through its properties of control and support for the voice has many roles. It supports both sung and spoken performance, it has a diagnostic role, it can offer an insight into an individual's physical and mental health, it can alert us to physiological changes associated with ageing and most of all it sustains life.

For those of us, whether in the field of clinical or artistic voice or in the fields of holistic and alternative health, the imperative is to provide the tools for those with whom we work to access their breath. Not only to access it but to use it to give them a voice with which to communicate, in the Editors' words, in ' a rich, complex and challenging world'.

EXERCISE

Title:	Exercise to encourage breath control
Aim:	To encourage and increase breath control.
Number of repetitions:	A maximum of four or five repetitions at one time, throughout the day. Make sure to allow time between repetitions in order to avoid hyperventilating.
Positioning:	Standing. If necessary begin by lying on the floor and then as proficiency increases, move to standing.

- Breathe in through your nose and out through your mouth, gently and easily, until a smooth and relaxed rhythm has been established.

- One you have achieved this, begin a silent count, breathing in for three seconds and out for three seconds.

- Maintain this silent count for several attempts and then begin to vary the length of the 'in' and 'out' breaths.

- Try a count of two for the 'in' breath and four for the 'out' breath.

- If you find it difficult to maintain the silent count while concentrating on the breath pattern, ask someone to count aloud for you.

- As you get better, decrease the 'in' breath time and increase the 'out' breath time. This more closely mirrors the pattern of breathing for sustained and controlled phonation.

- Breathe in on a count of two and this time out on/s/ for as long as possible but without strain.

- Make sure you do not allow any tension to occur in your lips, tongue or neck.

- If you do feel any tension occurring, reduce the length of time over which you maintain the /s/ sound.

BIBLIOGRAPHY

Andrews, M.L. (1995) *Manual of Voice Treatment*. San Diego: Singular Publishing Group.

Colton, R.H. and Casper, J.K. (1996) *Understanding Voice Problems*, 2nd edn. Baltimore: Williams & Wilkins.

Harris, T. (1992) 'The pharmacological treatment of voice disorders.' *Folia Phoniatrica*, pp. 143–54.

Hixon, T.J. (1987) *Respiratory Function in Speech and Song*. Boston: College Hill Press.

Koufman, J.A. (1998) 'What are Voice Disorders and Who Gets Them?' www.bgsm.edu?voice/voice-disorders. 22 November.

Martin, S. and Lockhart, M. (2000) *Working with Voice Disorders*. Bicester: Speechmark.

Martin, S and Lockhart, M. (2005) *The Voice Impact Profile*. Bicester: Speechmark.

Mathieson, L. (2001) *Greene & Mathieson's the Voice and its Disorders*, 6th edn. Chichester: Wiley Blackwell.

CHAPTER 3

Effects of Posture on Diaphragmatic Breath

APRIL PIERROT

WITH ILLUSTRATIONS BY TROY OHLSON

DEFINITIONS OF RESPIRATION

In the strictest sense, a definition of 'breath' might be simply the pulmonary exchange of gases upon which all of life undoubtedly depends, from its most rudimentary single cell manifestation to the enormously complex, multi-dimensional human form.

The human body, on every level, from single cell to total organism, is clearly unequivocal in its demand for breath. If we are to look properly, in minute detail, at the simple exchange of one gas for another, oxygen for carbon dioxide, (according to F. Matthias Alexander formulator of the principles of the Alexander Technique in the late nineteenth century) it will also be crucial to consider the entirety of the body's interconnected systems from gas exchange through to muscular function.

Conventional approaches to examining breath look to the anatomy and physiology of respiration. We see that it is a 'system'. As a broad view on the inhalation, the breath enters the body, flows through the lungs where the oxygen is taken into the blood stream, through the alveoli and transported around the body by the pump action of the heart muscle. Carbon dioxide is expelled from the blood by the muscularity of exhalation.

The organs of respiration, which comprise the respiratory 'system', are: the nose, the pharynx, the trachea, the bronchi, the bronchioles, the lungs and the alveoli. The physiological purpose of respiratory action is to introduce oxygen into the cells of the body through the blood and to expel carbon dioxide from the blood through the lungs. This is also known as the 'exchange of gases'.

Our 'impulse' to breathe is controlled by chemoreceptors in the aorta and carotid arteries, which are near the heart. These monitor levels of carbon dioxide and oxygen in the blood. When carbon dioxide levels are too high and oxygen too low, nerve impulses are sent by the medulla oblongata to the diaphragm telling it to contract, thus activating inhalation.

The primary muscles, those that activate and support the skeletal action that in turn allows inhalation and exhalation (in its fullest sense) to occur, are the diaphragm in conjunction with the intercostals, or inter rib, muscles.

Accessory muscles to respiration include the sternocleido mastoid muscles of the neck, the transversus abdominals, the scalenus, serratus posterior, pectorals, levatores costarum, transversus thoracis, quadratus lumborum and the deep muscles of the pelvic floor. Also necessary are the small muscles connected with the air passages controlling the size of the glottis, which is widened by inspiration at the laryngeal level and the laryngeal cartilages. These are also activated by the vagus nerve, which is deeply implicated in the work of the entire body.

The work of the diaphragm, discussed fully elsewhere in this book, is a muscular function. It is also an automatic function, determined by the medulla oblongata, which governs the inhalation and exhalation based on proprioceptive information from the bloodstream. The impulse for diaphragmatic movement is stimulated by the vagus nerve: it enervates the posterior portion of the external auditory canal and the eardrum and by anastomosis the larynx, the phrenic nerve and brancial nerves, which activate the upper shoulder girdle.

The vagus nerve is the longest and most variegated of cranial nerves. It originates in the cranium, as opposed to the spine and its name is derived from the Latin word meaning 'to wander'. The vagus nerve does wander, originating in the ear, innervating the heart, lungs and controlling the coronary nerve that in turn controls bronchial opening and closing and finally piercing the diaphragm on its way to the organs of the abdomen, which govern digestion and reproduction. Effective stimulation of vagus nerve fibres is what maintains the rhythm of respiration, as well as cardiac rhythms. Of course, we can and do alter our breathing rhythms consciously, but once our attention is diverted, it once again becomes the responsibility of the medulla oblongata.

Thus, on a purely anatomical level, we can appreciate the very close and synergistic relationship between the various mechanisms of the whole body, and most particularly of the heart, the lungs, the auditory and the vocal systems.

BODY AND BREATH SPEAK VOLUMES

Putting anatomy aside, we know ourselves as we do: we hear, we speak, we sing, we are moved on the heart level and the breath level. Our heart, our lungs, our voices may seize up with grief and fear. With voice and lungs: we gasp, we cry, we groan in pleasure and in grief. And at death, the breath rattles. Our vocal system, our hearts and lungs speak; likewise our whole body speaks volumes.

Even the vocabulary of breath tells us so much about its definite and refined role in psycho-physiology. We hold our breath when we are surprised, catch our breath in astonishment, we save our breath in not speaking where it will have no impact, and mutter under our breath in resentment. We give each other breathing space, and suffocate one another for want of it. The emotional state of anxious depression is characterized by sighing, arrhythmic breathing and high thoracic intake (see Chapter 2 by Stephanie Martin) and pain may be typified by sudden, sharp, gripping breath. We know all this, without being told; it is organic and a fully understood part of our experience. Whilst breath *can* be looked at from the purely physiological perspective of blood gases, if we look deeper we see the more sophisticated changes in neuro-function that foreshadow changes in breathing pattern.

Similarly, our bodily form or 'posture' is unconscious. It is part of our so-called and fully-formed 'identity'. Our posture is embodied attitude, unconscious and anatomical. It is that limiting unconscious anatomical mechanism which defines me as one thing with no possibility as another. What if we cannot fully feel the power of our own voices as a result of these limitations? What if after years of self-censoring, we end up with 'langues du bois', or 'tongues of wood' because that part of our muscularity, the tongue root, which has close muscular attachments to the vocal apparatus, has been so suppressed it has atrophied? What if we are unable to fully express ourselves emotionally because some part of our postural anatomy will not allow us? What will become of us? What does this mean for our potential to fully experience our own feelings, because they *are* embedded in our bodies, never mind to empathize with the feelings of others? And what if, in a proverbial slump, our bodies are deadened and our feelings likewise?

When we consider all this, we are beginning to consider the *entirety*. And why not? Without bodily form there can be no function, and without the need for function there would be no necessity for form. One is entirely and inextricably related to the other. Why should we not look to our form? It is the first thing we have, and perhaps all we will ever have. And in doing so, we may begin to understand so much more about ourselves than mere form and function will, on cursory examination, reveal? Closely observed, even a mechanistic approach can become a profound and very real starting point.

So, muscles attach to bone and bones are systemically arranged into skeletal form. We cannot, and should not, consider one without the other. Without skeletal form and functional muscularity there would be no respiration.

Here is where we begin: the body.

THE HEAD'S FUNCTIONAL RELATIONSHIP TO THE NECK AND BACK

If we want to influence or improve 'diaphragmatic action' in a profound and lasting way, one approach is to do this indirectly, with postural and vocal interventions. Is not voice an exhalation? Does the body not change shape on exhalation? If we alter our patterns of speech, or singing, will we not influence our breathing? If we alter our posture, will we not do likewise? Even without speaking or singing.

In the Alexander Technique, close and predominant attention is paid to:

- the balance of the skeletal parts

- the head's functional relationship to the neck and back

- the range of movement.

This range of movement encompasses:
- both the skeletal and the muscular

- from the top of the head to the atlanto occipital

- from the cervical to the lumbar spine to the ischial tuberosity

- from femur to foot.

Structural or skeletal alignment and its impact on muscular function, particularly respiratory or vocal function, is one of the cornerstones upon which the Alexander Technique was predicated.

The large muscular dome of the diaphragm with its flat central tendon, separates the thoracic cavity from the abdominal basin. It attaches at the lower end of the sternum, at the underside of the xyphoid process on the front of the body, to the lowest six ribs on either side and to the first three lumbar vertebrae at the back by two muscular crura. The crura are arranged vertically, on the inside of spine, and assist in pulling down the diaphragm on inhalation. It weaves fibrously into the belly of the transverse abdominal muscles, and indeed into the thoracic and abdominal organs such as the liver.

Furthermore, the crura of the diaphragm have important fibrous connections to the hip flexors, the psoas major and the iliacus.

During inhalation, the diaphragm is sensitized to contract, flattening and creating a vacuum, thus air is pulled into the lungs. As the diaphragm flattens, it displaces the abdominal organs downwards and outwards. The tummy, or more correctly, the organs of the pelvic basin displace. As the surface area of the lungs expands, putting pressure on the intercostal muscles, they respond by pivoting the ribs upwards and forwards, increasing the diameter of the chest and pulling air into the lungs to equalize pressure. Thus, there is a synergistic muscularity between the diaphragm, the abdominals and the intercostalmuscles that facilitate inhalation.

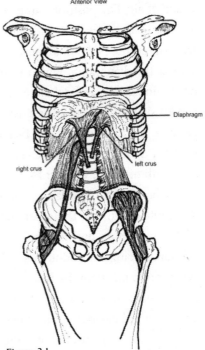

Figure 3.1

In exhalation, the opposite occurs. The abdominals contract slightly, pushing the diaphragm which moves upwards into its original dome shape, impinging up into the chest cavity and reducing the chest area volume, causing the air to be expelled. If the breath line on exhalation is lengthened, as for instance in singing or very demanding vocal work, the abdominal contraction will eventually begin to tug on the bottom of the pelvis, or pubic bone.

PELVIC ALIGNMENT

Western bodywork and vocal traditions, recognizing the importance of the pelvic alignment to respiration and indeed to controlled and easeful function, may crudely 'correct' the pelvic alignment by pushing down the 'tailbones', or tucking under the pelvis. To accomplish this, one can try a number of strategies, tensing the gluteuls, tightening the abdominal wall, drawing down on the hip flexors or collapsing the lumbar spine. But unfortunately while any of these strategies may correct the pelvic or lumbar alignment in a superficial sense, it also prevents the very synergistic movement of the muscles of the pelvis and rib cage during breath work which we are ideally seeking to promote.

If the position of the lumbar spine is compromised, the displacement of the abdominal organs on inhalation will be impeded and will therefore act to diminish the intake of air. The position can be compromised by being either too far forward as in lordosis, exaggerated lumbar curve, or too far back, as happens in postural slumping. Likewise, if the abdominal muscles are tense, the abdominal organs will be forced up against the diaphragm, which in turn will not be able to properly move downward during inhalation and exhalation.

All skeletal movement is predicated on expansion or contraction of antagonistic muscles. For example, as my bicep contracts, my triceps lengthen and my forearm moves. I do not have to engineer this. I have only to think of the movement and the body will organize the rest for me.

In breathing, the diaphragm and abdominal muscles must act as antagonists, when one lengthens, the other shortens; thus accomplishing the desired movement of the diaphragm during inhalation and exhalation. If the lumbar spine is in contraction, forcing the abdominal muscles into release and the intercostal muscles into extension to maintain the concomitant rib posture, how can the abdominals properly support exhalation and the ribs further swing on inhalation? The body will prioritize structural balance at the expense of function. Both the head and the neck act as accessories to respiration, but if the head is off balance and thus, also, the muscles of the neck, then they are busy maintaining uprightness, so how can they be properly concerned with breathing?

In addition to this, if as a result of incomplete function the oxygen and carbon dioxide exchange is incomplete, this will in turn affect the acid and alkaline balance in the blood, promoting an overall muscular tetany, or contraction of voluntary muscle. So, it is easily a vicious circle.

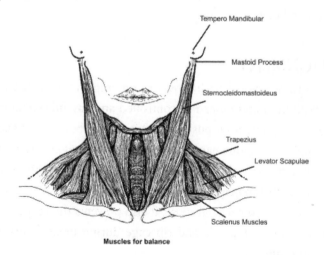

Figure 3.2

STRUCTURAL BALANCE

As we have seen, while it may be said that the most important *muscle* for breathing is the diaphragm, from the point of view of Alexander Technique the most important component in breathing is the skeletal balance between head, the neck, the cervical spine, the fully lengthened thoracic and lumbar spine and the pelvis and leg. It is the resultant *equilibrium* of the skeletal weight, and the resultant placement of emphasis in the pelvis, that produces a balanced muscularity in breathing (i.e. full diaphragmatic breath). Say what you will, no end of breathing into the back or the abdomen or indeed the ribs will accomplish inherently well-organized breath work. Once you stop thinking about it, your body will go back to doing what it is programmed skeletally to do.

The balance of the whole body, 'the posture' should be the first focus of attention. In placing hands on and applying upward direction to the spine, the Alexander teacher 'forces' the body to *experience* the correct relationships between legs, pelvis, spine, shoulder girdle and head, the balance of which is crucial to full breath. Thus, one learns *kinaesthetically* the correct influence of skeletal posture on breathing and the most advantageous muscular tone.

Having understood all this, now we can look in more detail, by attempting some practical exercises, which might illustrate the deeper functions of diaphragmatic breathing as it relates to an integrated skeletal system.

PRACTICAL EXERCISES
Wall exercises
Exercise 1: Standing against the wall

Title: Sliding the back down the wall

Aim: To explore the synergistic relationship between the legs, the lumbar and the head/neck/back in movement

- Stand with your back to the wall, as in Figure 3.3.

- Allow your feet to be hip width apart, with a slight turn out on the feet. Heels should be 5–7 cm away from the wall, weight evenly distributed on both feet.

- Focus the attention forward, allow the eyes to soft gaze and notice the effect on the neck, nose and mouth.

- Allow your knees to start to move out and over your toes and at the same time imagine that your back is providing the impulse to move.

- Give yourself the direction to slide the back to the wall.

- Give your back the instruction to remain lengthened, but at the same time slide in space down the wall. Thus we are directing up in the spine, but moving down in space at the same time. This is an important instruction. We want to have the spatial direction. It is the *movement in space which is important*, not an instruction to any particular muscle in the body. The body will interpret it in an appropriate fashion if the preconditions are good.

- Notice the pelvis tilting in response to the instruction and the lumbar spine releasing backwards as you slide down the wall.

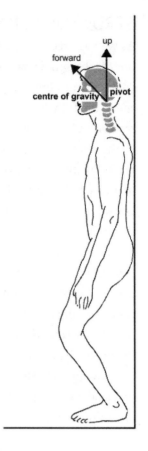

Figure 3.3

Comments

These concomitant changes are important to notice, as they are inter-related. The relationship between the legs, pelvis and lumbar spine provide a great deal of information kinaesthetically about this part of the body and its importance for respiration.

Exercise 2: Breath and head direction

Title: Balancing the head on top of the shoulder girdle

Aim: To understand how breath is influenced by the relationship between the head the neck and the shoulder girdle

- Allow the head to rest softly on top of the shoulders with the face forward: forward and up.

- Balance the head on top of lengthened spine.

- Lengthen and widen the back: from hips to cranium.

- Allow the muscles at the back of the neck to be free, at the same time make sure the neck is in full extension. Do not over lengthen the neck.

- Allow the clavicles to release away into the shoulder joint.

- Allow the head weight to relax forward.

- Allow the shoulder blades to relax down into the back.

- Notice what happens to the breath. Notice the relationship of our 'posture' in this position to our breath.

To observe a contrasting 'posture':
- Tip the head back, contracting the muscles at the back of the neck and notice what happens to the air as it enters into the nostrils.

- Notice what happens to the ribs on both inhalation and exhalation.

Comments

So, the movement of the ribs (the breath) alters in relationship to the position of the head and the condition of the spine (in particular the cervical spine, or the neck).

Continuation
- Return to lengthening the spine and releasing the neck. Let the weight of the head nod forward until the neck, as the back of the body lengthens.

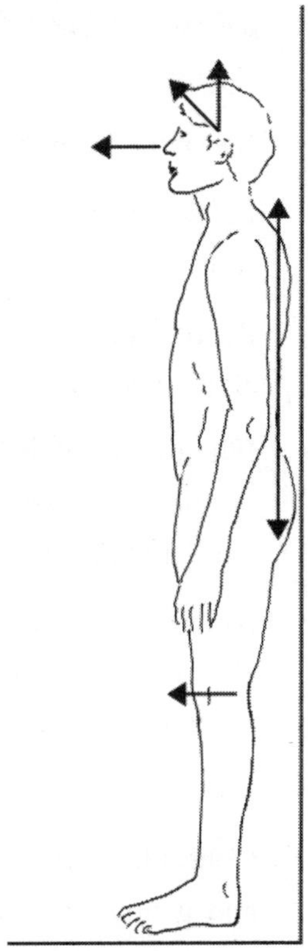

Figure 3.4

- Notice how this allows the nostrils to release into inhalation and the larynx to relax in the 'neck'. (The larynx softens into position in the front of the neck.)

- Note the relationship between the head direction, back of the neck release and the relaxing of the larynx.

Exercise 3: Sternum/ribs placement

Title: Exploring the Lumbar/Ribcage/Sternum placement
Aim: To understand how the lumbar/rib/sternum relationship impacts on respiration
- Still standing against the wall, pull up on the upper rib cage and sternum.

- Notice how this 'posture' affects your breath.

- Notice the change in the position of the lumbar spine. Feel the affect of the upper clavicular breath and consequently hyperventilation.

Compare and contrast

- Release the base of the sternum (xyphoid process) into the abdominal wall above the navel.

- Relax the sternum.

- Relax the base of the ribs at the point that the rib base embeds into the abdominal wall.

- Relax (but do not collapse) the sternum. Keep the sternum released into the abdominals (without tension) and notice the way the ribs fill out.

- Inhale and exhale fully, but keep the spine lengthened. Do not collapse the spine on the exhalation and notice how the maintaining of 'upright' posture allows for a fuller exhalation.

- Notice the 'elastic' recoil of the lungs on the in-breath. The mechanical effectiveness of the in-breath is dependent on the free length of spine, as well as the unencumbered width of ribs.

- Breathe again.

- Concentrate your breath on maintaining the spinal length at the same time as and gently encouraging (with your thought) the already existing frontal reflex movement of the ribs on inhalation/exhalation.

Exercise 4: Jaw opening/whispered 'AH' and 'SA'

Title: The whispered 'AH'
Aim: To release the jaw and open the space for the breath

- Place your index finger at the little indentation in front of the small piece of cartilage in front of the opening to the ear.

- Sink your index finger into this opening and next, open your jaw. Feel the action of the temporo mandibular joint.

- Repeat the tipping back of the head and the opening of the jaw. Notice the difference.

- Let the head weight nod forward, allowing the larynx to relax.

- Imagine you are about to yawn, but 'say no' to yawning. Don't yawn, but instead notice what happens in the nostrils, the glottal opening, the soft palate and the larynx, the clavicles, sternum and ribs.

- Imagine yawning, inhale through the nostrils and exhale making an 'unvoiced' 'AH' sound.

- Notice the relationship of the exhalation and the reflex movement of both the abdomen and the ribs.

- This time make an unvoiced 'SA' sound.

- Notice the difference in the behaviour of the abdomen when we ask ourselves to say 'SA' as opposed to 'AH'.

- Tip over the hips, maintaining the length of the spine. This is the Position of Mechanical Advantage (Monkey).

- Allow the breath to continue, and notice the freedom of movement when the lumbar spine is uncompromised.

Exercise 5: Rib cage/pelvis alignment

Title: Monkey

Aim: To find the proper balance of weight and muscularity in the pelvic basin, thus freeing the rib cage to move with respiration

- In Monkey, notice the relationship between base of ribs, lumbar spine and pelvis.

- Imagine an integrating line from base of lateral ribs to hip joints.

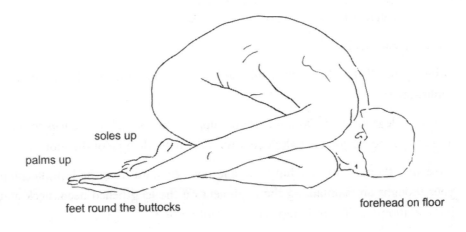

soles up

palms up

feet round the buttocks

forehead on floor

Figure 3.5

- Be aware of the relationship of iliac crests to lumbar spine/rib cage.

- The rib cage is skeletally very light. Any intercostal or abdominal tension means the rib movement will be impeded and therefore the breath can easily be compromised.

Floor exercise
Exercise: Hip pelvic placements

Title: Child's Pose

Aim: To understand how tension in the hip/lumbar region can impede the lengthening of the spine and full diaphragmatic breath

- Take the position illustrated in Figure 3.5; this is called Child's Pose in yoga.

- Notice where the hip joints are.

- Tense the hips; notice the effect on the abdominal wall and on the breath.

- Release in the hip joints and notice the effect on your breath.

- Notice that tensing the hips narrows the distance between femur and pelvis and affects breathing because the psoas muscles are shortening. When the psoas releases, the spine extends and lengthens, releasing the breath.

Chair exercise
Exercise: Sitting in chair: forward flexion on exhalation

Title: Exploring the hip/pelvis alignment and the deep muscularity of the pelvis

Aim: To understand the relationship between the hips and the alignment of the pelvis and how this impacts on the breath

- Sit in a comfortable chair.

- Bring yourself to the very edge and sit up on your sit bones (ischial tuburosities).

- Relax the legs forward. Do not tense the upper limb, but allow the legs to relax away from the hip joints in alignment with the natural angle of the foot.

- Take your thought into the hip joint, and pivot forward from the hips, keeping your thought on maintaining the alignment on the lengthened head, neck and back relationship. Think in terms of line, not tension.

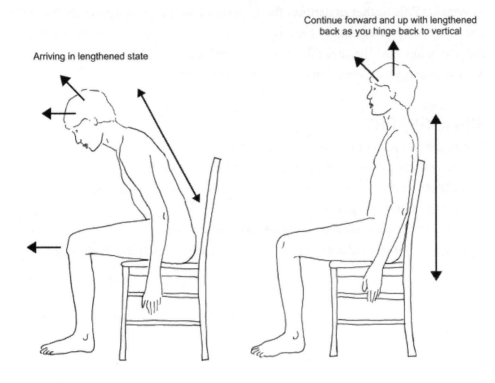

Figure 3.6

- Balance the line from the head to the hips, but think about activating the movement from the hips.

- Notice what muscles do the work. The muscles of the pelvis basin balance the work.

- Notice that as we use these deep muscles, which attach the lumbar to the legs as well as controlling the pelvis weight, the upper body releases and the shoulders relax into the back.

- Notice that when we are habituated to activate the muscles of the pelvis, the legs and the upper body tend to release.

CONCLUSION

We can see, overall, that the respiratory system is very dependant on the full co-ordinated action of the muscularity of the pelvis and of properly aligned skeletal movement. This further underlines the importance of a holistic approach, exemplified in work by practitioners such as F.M. Alexander, in order to provide a key to understanding how the skeletal, neuro-chemical and muscular systems of the body work in synergy to accomplish optimal respiratory function.

BIBLIOGRAPHY

Gray, H. (1993) *Gray's Anatomy*. Stevenage: Magpie Books Ltd.

Ellis, H. (1992) *Clinical Anatomy* (FRCS 6th Edition). Blackwell Scientific Press

Todd, Mabel E. (1937) *The Thinking Body* unabridged edition. Princeton Book Company

McCallion, M. (1988) *The Voice Book*. London: Faber and Faber

Blandine C. (1993) *Anatomy of Movement*. Seattle, WA: Eastland Press

Udupa, K.N. (1978) *Stress and Its Management by Yoga* (5th Edition). New Delhi: Motilal Publications

CHAPTER 4

The Art of Breathing

JESSICA WOLF

Breathing is indispensable. It is as fundamental to life as the beating of our heart. Because we usually take breathing for granted, we tend not to realize the harmful effects that faulty breathing can have on us, or the freedom we can gain by improving how we breathe. Breathing, involuntary in nature, is something we can influence. Most of us begin life breathing fully and without strain. For many reasons, our natural breathing abilities and rhythms become compromised as we move through life.

For the past 30 years, I have been helping people restore their natural breathing patterns using a method I have developed called 'The Art of Breathing.'[1] It is based upon the work of F.M. Alexander (who invented the technique that bears his name) and Carl Stough.

For those of you not familiar with it, the Alexander Technique is a simple and proven method of self-care which increases ease of movement and alleviates pain and stress caused by everyday misuse of the body. It is unique among all the psychophysical techniques because it is the only one that can make changes that will last a lifetime. Less known is that Alexander's original discovery was specifically about the respiratory system. In his time, Alexander became known as 'the breathing man'.

The signature idea of the Alexander Technique is this: how we 'use' our bodies affects how we function; therefore, misuse causes malfunction. We all have unconscious movement habits, and habit is powerful. Often it is *how* we do something that creates the problem, not the activity itself. Many people are mystified by their back

---

1   The 'Art of Breathing' is a phrase Alexander coined to originally name his technique in 1903

pain, excess tension or other physical symptoms. You often hear people say, 'My breathing never gave me any problems before', or 'I must be getting older'. These conditions don't just happen; they develop over time – like a train coming around a bend: you can't see it at first, but it's coming.

F.M. Alexander (1869–1955) was a Shakespearean actor famous for his dramatic recitations, but during performances he would grow hoarse. Doctors advised him to rest his voice, but as soon as he began to use it again, the problem returned. To end the hoarseness once and for all, he started observing himself, looking for behaviour that might have caused his vocal difficulties. He noticed that at the moment of speaking, he would stiffen his neck, raise his shoulders and unconsciously gasp for breath. This pattern caused compression along his spine, constriction in his throat, and a gasping sound during inhalation.

Alexander recognized that in order to heal, he needed to stop the unnecessary effort he had been using to make sound. To prevent this counter-productive activity, he would have to focus on the *whole* of himself. He would need to learn to support himself from the ground up, and find a new balance for his head in order to allow the muscles of his neck, chest and shoulders to be at ease. Once this wholeness was achieved, he didn't need to 'muscle' individual parts. He also found it increased his breathing capacity. Alexander said: 'Breath is the life; and breathing capacity is the measure of life'[2] (Alexander 1995, p. 22).

At about the time Alexander died, another man was making significant contributions to the field of breathing. Carl Stough (1926–2000), a modern-day pioneer in the science of respiration, identified a particular coordination that allows the respiratory system to function at maximum efficiency with minimum effort. He called this 'breathing coordination'.[3] Stough's specialized knowledge was the result of years of musical training, choral conducting and work with patients with emphysema (a debilitating and irreversible respiratory disease). Patients with respiratory illness spend their lives trying to get an adequate breath. But it wasn't just ill patients who had this problem. Stough observed that anyone from the fit athlete to the skilled performer could also suffer from a loss of natural breathing coordination.

He stated: 'Breathing Coordination is breathing in that individual pattern which engages all the muscles of respiration, both voluntary and involuntary and provides the most efficient deflation and inflation of the lungs with the least amount of effort' (Stough 1970, p. 26). Stough discovered a way to facilitate breathing coordination, by using a set of simple procedures that reestablish normal, involuntary breathing.

---

2   Quoted from *The Prevention and Cure of Consumption* (1903) Alexander, F.M. (1995) Articles and Lectures. London: Mouritz.

3   'breathing coordination' is the name given by Carl Stough to describe the exact way the respiratory system was designed to function at maximum efficiency with minimum effort.

Imagine the benefits of this work: developing physical freedom, releasing tension, restoring mobility to overworked muscles, gaining access to the breath and revealing pathways to emotional release. I use both the Alexander Technique and Stough's Principles of Breathing Coordination when I teach the actors in my classes at the Yale School of Drama and the people (actors and non-actors alike) whom I see in my private practice.

I often begin my workshops for the public or classes for actors and singers with some guided imagery. I refer to it as a 'breathing meditation' and it is meant to awaken their senses. The image I use that best captures 'The Art of Breathing' is the movement of the ocean – its ebb and flow, the inevitability of the waves.

> Imagine yourself by the sea. Feel the moist air on your skin, taste the salt on your lips; smell the ocean's breeze. Look and listen to the ongoing motion of the waves. The waves break; some are huge and have a tremendous impact as they crash onto the beach. Others may swoosh in rhythmical phrasing as they reach the shore and recede. And then there are the small waves which simply lap along the shore, sometimes coming in one right after the next. We can look out at the ocean, sometimes several hundred yards from the beach, and sense a stillness in the water. Lo and behold, the quiet changes and a wave begins to build; it reaches its crescendo, breaks on the sand and joins the ocean's water again. Waves continue to form, they move in and out, each with its own rhythm and impact, and never will they be repeated.

The involuntary nature of our breath has the same quality. Breath is an ongoing motion. We never have to worry about our next breath. Some breaths may be huge, changing the entire circumference of the body. Movement of breath may be experienced in the chest, the belly, the shoulders, the pelvis and the back. When the breath moves out, the entire three-dimensional torso changes shape.

Some breaths may accelerate, some may feel like you are sipping tiny bits of air. Nothing is mechanical, and the less you interfere with the involuntary nature of the breath, the easier it is to have the breath return. Breath changes from moment to moment, but you never have to do anything to make this happen. Like the ocean's waves, the breath that has just moved out will never be repeated. Each breath is authentic, each new breath in is in response to the breath that just moved out.

Could you consider that you never have to 'take' another breath? Breathing is something that happens for you, to you. There is no need to *do* anything[4]. Simply let your breath out and now notice the return of the breath. A new breath will arrive.

---

4   'You don't need to do anything You are undoing rather than doing' Jessica Wolf (2004) Notes from a lecture. Yale School of Drama.

Unfortunately, such ease is often not the case. In today's world, respiratory complications can arrive from a myriad of causes: pollution, stress, neuromuscular and skeletal problems, illness such as asthma, headache, gastrointestinal problems, and last but not least, emotional problems. Increasingly, people are being diagnosed with symptoms of anxiety and depression and are treated with prescription medication. In such cases, the medication causes drowsiness, a dulling of the senses and has a similar effect on the respiratory system.

Postural problems often restrict breathing which, in turn, limits the turnover of air and decreases our general mobility. People complain of not being able to 'take a breath' or of not having a satisfying breath. A collapse of the chest can cause the breath to feel shallow and evoke an emotional sensation of depression, without our realizing it. Similarly, stiffening to 'stand up straight' can lead to feelings of anxiety and stress.

Most of us are not able to leave ourselves alone and let the breathing *do* itself. We've acquired all sorts of ways to limit the ease of our breath. The challenge, then, is to eliminate the habits that interfere with natural, involuntary breathing.

To better understand how patterns of misuse can compromise a human being, I will tell you the story of one of my acting students. For an actor, there is nothing more essential than the breath, and the problems that arise when it is interfered with. I hope this will be instructive for performers and non-performers alike.

Case study: Sophie

Sophie, a 35 year-old professional actor, came to me concerned about her voice. She had been working professionally in Broadway theatres for seven years and had just been cast in a production at Lincoln Center. As Sophie endured the demands of rehearsal and performance, she found it increasingly difficult to be heard. Her efforts to project her voice became excruciating, and she began to despair about fulfilling the role she had so eagerly sought. This was more than a technical problem; it impaired Sophie's ability to communicate and to access her emotions. Her career depended on this performance, so the stakes were high and she was desperate to solve her problem. And her problem wasn't confined to the professional sphere. Even her social life was threatened: when meeting friends in restaurants, she strained to be heard over ambient noise.

When we first started working together, Sophie was surprised that I didn't focus on her voice. But her voice wasn't the problem; it was a manifestation of the problem. As F.M. Alexander put it, 'Nature does not work in parts; she treats everything as a whole' (Alexander 1995, p. 41). Unfortunately, many people focus on the symptom but they fail to see its cause. Sophie's vocal problems were inextricably linked to faulty breathing patterns, which in turn related to improper use of her body as a whole. We began by working on her overall movement pattern in order to restore her natural connection to her breath, applying the principles that Alexander discovered in restoring his own voice.

At the outset, I wanted to make Sophie aware of how she was interfering with her coordination. It was a case of faulty sensory awareness: when we think we are doing something very different from what we are actually doing. A glance in a mirror or a store window often reveals that we are standing quite differently from how we imagine. And on a deeper level, we may also have very wrong ideas about how our internal system actually works. I often tell my students it is essential that they become intimately familiar with their bodies.

In Sophie's case, I found that her concept of how her respiratory system functioned was quite inaccurate. She knew that the diaphragm is the primary muscle of respiration, but she didn't understand how it functioned nor where it was located. Yet this understanding is crucial; the diaphragm is the foundation of the entire respiratory system. Sophie thought she was doing a good thing by breathing 'diaphragmatically' – when, in fact, all Sophie was doing by breathing this way was pushing her abdominal muscles forward. What is often understood as 'diaphragmatic breathing' is not something to aspire to.

The diaphragm is an involuntary muscle/organ; we don't have direct control over it. (Like the heart, its movement is controlled by the autonomic system.) When the diaphragm descends on an inhale, it naturally causes the abdomen to move outward – not because you are filling your abdomen with air (there is no lung in the belly!), but because the diaphragm is compressing your internal organs. So the very concept of 'diaphragmatic breathing' also called 'belly breathing' is erroneous. In fact, habitual pushing the belly out on the inhale weakens the diaphragm, so that it becomes incapable of its full range of movement, and full exhalation and inhalation become impossible.

Another interfering breathing habit is 'accessory' breathing; that is, over activating one's chest, shoulder and neck muscles to breathe. Both accessory breathing and belly breathing result in a neglect of the back. If the back muscles are not well coordinated, the abdominal muscles will pull down on the spine and cause a collapse in the lower back. The ribs will lose their mobility and there will be a decrease in lung capacity, which can lead to loss of the voice and chronic back and neck pain. If the reaction to these difficulties is to push and pull the abdominals in and out to breathe, the spine collapses even more. Thus, one bad habit triggers another.

I asked Sophie to speak some of her text. I could see and hear that she was overworking her abdominals and not breathing efficiently. Without realizing it, her breathing habits were obscuring and limiting her ability to communicate and express herself, and interfering with her intuitive rhythm. Additionally, the excess effort she was using to 'muscle' her abdominals (belly breathing) was creating tension in her entire body.

In order for Sophie to deliver the performance she was capable of, we needed to return her breath to its natural involuntary state, freeing her to express her full vocal and emotional palette. I explained to Sophie that she didn't have to do anything to breathe; the diaphragm knows what to do. In Alexander's terms, she could learn to inhibit[5] her habitual over-exertion to make way for the natural process. Simply stated, she needed to get out of her own way.

When I first observed Sophie, she was pulling her head in a manner that Alexander called 'back and down': lifting her chin, pressing the back of her skull down, compressing her neck. This is a widespread pattern, the same one that Alexander observed in himself. Through his long process of self-experiment, he came to realize that this back and down pressure restricts space in the throat and interferes with reflexive, harmonious breathing. In Sophie's case, as in many others, this characteristic head/neck relationship made her back and chest rigid.

I asked Sophie to notice her standing posture. Immediately she observed that she locked her knees. As we explored the possibility of balancing more easily on supple legs, Sophie made an unexpected connection: to the base of her tongue. As she released her knees, she released her jaw. That led to a release of her tongue, and she felt more space inside her mouth. Her insight revealed exactly what I wanted to convey: that the overall coordination of the body determines the functioning of the breath and the voice. We were both thrilled by her discovery.

Using the delicate Alexander touch that allows the teacher to both sense and suggest subtle shifts in the student's body, I guided Sophie into a freer, more dynamic alignment, with her head balanced forward and up on her spine. This new head/neck relationship caused a shift in her foundation. Sophie released her weight down through her feet and began to sense the floor. She literally stopped holding herself up. We both laughed about her curious pattern of pressing down on the back of her tongue, as if that could help her stand. Sophie's frozen energy began to thaw; a lovely quality of ease came over her.

When Sophie returned for her lesson the following week, she was in good spirits. She said that her body awareness during rehearsal had improved. Since high heels were part of her costume, she knew that it would take attention to avoid stiffening her legs. Because the diaphragm attaches at the lower spine and the muscles in the legs also connect up into the back, when we brace in our legs we interfere with our breath. Efficient posture is critical for efficient breathing.

---

5   In the Alexander Technique, 'inhibition' is a mindful skill used to prevent habitual or unwanted behaviour as it is about to begin or as it is happening.

It was then time to focus on Sophie's torso by doing 'table work' – that is, with Sophie lying on her back on a padded table. Because it is difficult to trust a new coordination, it's easier for the student to learn lying down, without fighting the effects of gravity. Sophie would then be able to use this improved coordination when she was more active in her daily life. I also encouraged Sophie to practise lying down on her own, in what I call 'active rest'.[6] Time spent lying down helps a person release the muscular tension that builds throughout the day, gently re-establishes connection among all parts of the body and consequently encourages improved breathing.

As I guided Sophie with a light manual touch and verbal cues, I could sense the underlying pressure in her torso. Her shoulders and ribs felt stiff; but her belly felt even tighter, hindering her breath. I sensed that her habit of holding and strain was originating in her abdomen. I asked if she noticed any connection between her belly and her throat. Immediately she responded that her tongue and jaw felt locked.

As Stough noted: 'All the muscles of breathing were intended to operate in a synergistic pattern with the stress of the work load distributed evenly among them' (Stough 1970, p. 156). Stough found that this coordination could be developed using a long and relaxed exhalation. I encouraged Sophie to think along the length of her spine while breathing out. I asked her to effortlessly flap the tongue in a silent 'la, la, la'. Stough used this method to promote a complete exhalation and a natural, reflexive inhalation in response (all while enabling the throat to stay open). A longer, relaxed exhalation removes more stale air from the lungs, thus making more room for air to return.

Once Sophie had learned to release her breath without muscling, she was ready to make sound. We started by counting to five aloud and then continued counting silently until the completion of the exhalation. Once the new breath arrived, we increased the count to ten aloud and again finished by silently counting to the breath's conclusion. Like the silent 'la', this gradually increasing audible count extends the exhalation, so that the next inhalation feeds in a greater volume of air. I told Sophie never to misjudge the reason for the count. There is no prescribed number to reach on the exhale; that would destroy natural breathing and replace it with forced patterns. Breathing is a rhythmical function; it is not mechanical.

During this process, if I felt Sophie's lower abdomen tensing, I would know that she was forcing her breath and would ask her to go back to the silent 'la' as a way to return to her relaxed exhale. I was teaching her body to use an

---

6 'Active rest' is a semi-supine position lying on your back with your knees bent. Books are placed under your head to give it support and to allow the muscles of your neck to lengthen. As you rest for at least 10 minutes a day, you become aware of yourself. Notice yourself; your body and your breath. Let the tension release. Jessica Wolf (1999) Notes from a class. Yale School of Drama.

appropriate amount of tension. Although I am not in favour of voluntary 'muscling', muscle tension itself is not the villain; it is necessary to function. Well-coordinated amounts of muscular energy must be available and responsive to the constantly changing needs of the body and voice.

As I worked with Sophie in this manner, I asked her to imagine the breath fueling the length of her spine; she was to 'do' nothing more than to think of her breath moving as she directed her spine to release into length. I encouraged Sophie to think of her torso as a three-dimensional container. This would remind her to include her back in her thought. Most functions of the respiratory system occur higher and deeper in the body than we generally realize. The top of our lungs reach up in front under the collarbone, and the mass of our lungs extend down into the back of the body. Remember where your doctor listens to your breathing first? The stethoscope is placed on your back. It is for this reason that we must include the whole of the torso and encourage breathing to function three dimensionally – all the way around, not just in front as many people imagine. But again, I was not asking Sophie to 'do' anything; rather, she was to bring her attention to her back and be aware of its capacity to move as she breathed. This awareness, properly cultivated, is enough to cause the muscles of the torso to release appropriately. As Sophie's back expanded, I found new mobility in her ribs. Then her abdomen and chest released. Sophie experienced the ongoing motion of her breath. She commented on its spontaneity and recognized its potent connection to her thoughts and feelings.

During another lesson, we worked on the procedure F.M. Alexander called 'the whispered ah', an exercise used to prepare for speaking.[7] Whispering is not something that we normally do, so we have fewer ingrained habits that might interfere with the breath. In addition, Alexander believed that a whisper could reveal faulty vocal habits that speaking aloud obscured. If the whispered 'ah' is done incorrectly, the throat constricts (contributing to already existing tension in the throat) and causes facial muscles to strain. Done correctly, it supports the head, neck and back relationship.

Beginning with an exhalation, Sophie whispered the 'ah' vowel as she allowed her whole torso to lengthen and widen. She let her jaw open without pulling her head back and down. Rather than voluntarily muscling the exhale, Sophie let go of her rigid ribs and tight belly. Her body expanded and the whisper was released. Again I began to feel motion along the spine and mobility in her ribs. This was very encouraging to Sophie, as she experienced the benefits of an overall coordination and a sense of well-being.

We then played with singing the 'ah' vowel sound. She sustained the 'ah' without effort. The whole of Sophie resonated with her impulse to speak. She

7   'The whispered ah' is an exercise in coordination. Alexander began the breathing cycle with exhalation which was followed by the return of the breath, the inhalation. Jessica Wolf (1999) Notes from a lecture. Integrative Healthcare of Symposium.

said she felt as if 'the sound was spinning out her ears'. Rather than muscling, Sophie allowed time and internal space for the air to arrive. 'Just thinking about my body,' she said, 'and imagining the internal movement of my breath makes it easier for me to breathe.' As she spoke about the healing effect of awareness, I could hear more vitality in her voice.

Over a period of many weeks in which Sophie had a dozen lessons, she learned to apply her newly acquired skills to the act of speaking. With her new-found breathing coordination, she was now hearing the depth, truth and full-ness of her voice. The diaphragm is not just a pump that brings air in and out of the lungs; it is a great organ of expression. Sophie experienced her breath as actually moving her thought and emotion. She said she had always heard about psycho-physical change, but for the first time she recognized something new. 'When my breath changed, I changed.'

The play had a very successful, long run. When it closed in New York City, Sophie remained with the company and went on the road for another six months. She was mindful of herself and careful to do her lying-down work (active rest) which included specific 'exhalation études'[8] (like the silent 'la' and counting). Expressing herself, on stage and in life, was no longer a problem. She remained aware of the old habits that interfered with her voice, and was able to substitute new patterns of use with self-confidence.

As the result of Sophie's learning process, she had acquired tools to free her from the constraints of artificial breath control and breath support. This return to ease and release of the breath, body and voice is a slow process, but well worth the joy and the journey.

Case study: Edward in pain

Two years ago I received a phone call from Edward, a 51-year-old partner in a law firm, who told me his chronic headaches had become so intense that he could no longer do his job. He had consulted doctors, taken medication and tried physical therapy – none of which seemed to be helping him to feel bet-ter. He was desperate to find lasting relief and had taken a leave of absence to give himself time to heal. He recalled a friend of his telling him about a technique that dealt with back pain, headaches and breath. Ordinarily Edward

---

8   'Exhaltation études' is a phrase I use when I teach singers and instrumentalists. These procedures may be practised during active rest, chair work and as you go about warming up for rehearsal and performance. Jessica Wolf (1999) Notes from a lecture. Aspen Music Festival.

regarded such 'alternative healing techniques' with scepticism, but pain – the great motivator – led Edward to come and see me anyway.

Edward had accumulated decades of unconscious bad habits that restricted his body's mobility and interfered with his breath. By the time he came to me, Edward had lost a lot of flexibility and thus had very few choices in his overall movement. His hips were locked onto his legs; his neck and shoulders were held so tight that he strained when he turned his head; his voice was meek; and he was frustrated by his chronic pain.

Edward wasn't just suffering from headaches. He had essentially been stuck in a fight or flight response for years. His headaches were the acute stress response to being trapped in this physical and energetic state. This prolonged stress had taken its toll on Edward's body and mind. He was exhausted. His life was extremely pressured for a variety of reasons and he had no 'downtime', no recuperation. Edward was constantly wired. He said: 'I feel like my breath and my heartbeat just accelerate out of nowhere, for no reason.' It was a real statement of concern. He was frightened by these sensations.

And he was right to be frightened, because his overall well-being was in jeopardy. When people are in pain, they move less; and when they move less, their muscles start to atrophy and their bodies get weaker – which in turn compromises their respiratory and circulatory systems. Edward's headache was not the problem; it was a manifestation of the problem. I knew using the principles of the Alexander Technique could help diffuse the emotional and physical problems that Edward was experiencing in his life.

Instead of focusing on the symptom we agreed to search for the cause. The first step in Edward's healing process would be for him to become aware of how his psycho-physical habits were causing his headaches. During his long working hours, the ways he slouched as he spoke to clients, slumped at a desk, bent his ear into the phone and hunched his back toward his computer to read a brief were exacerbating his already existing pain. Mis-use in one part of the body triggers mis-use in another part. Pain begets pain. So it was important for Edward to acquire a sense of the whole self – mind and body – as we consciously explored his condition and his responses to the pain.

During weekly lessons with Edward, I would give verbal instruction and gentle, 'hands-on' guidance to help restore his body's natural ease and coordination. I was looking to resolve Edward's postural and functional problems that were undermining his comfort, productivity and overall health. As I identified several patterns of movement that seemed to be aggravating his pain, he was able to recognize these postures and the effect they had on him. For example, we observed his habit of sinking his pelvis down onto his legs while standing. As we explored how he could balance more easily on his legs and feet, Edward made an unexpected connection to his upper body. When he released his hips, he let go of his neck and was immediately impressed with the release of tension in his chest. He realized that by really using his legs to stand (that is, by releasing the weight of his body through his legs onto his feet and into the ground), he didn't have to contract his torso to stand (that is, by lifting his shoulders, clenching his buttocks and tightening his belly). He immediately perceived this as a great way to reduce tension. Soon, he was able to track the differences in the two patterns and could choose to stand for longer periods of time without discomfort.

Within a month of taking lessons, Edward discovered another significant habit that contributed to his pain. I asked him to observe how he was sitting; to notice the shape of his body and how it might be affecting his breathing pattern.

Edward observed that, when sitting, he collapsed his upper body forward and sunk in his chest. He suddenly exclaimed: 'I'm jutting my neck forward and pulling my head back. And I'm holding my breath!'

The importance of respiratory re-education is crucial to regaining natural coordination of breath, body and mind. In fact, many physical problems – and emotional distress as well – are the result of insufficient oxygen, caused by faulty respiratory patterns. Edward's breathing coordination had been disturbed by years of fatigue and stress. He had become so accustomed to holding his breath, that his breathing was no longer rhythmical or reflexive. In order to reawaken Edward's respiratory system, we had to redevelop his breathing coordination. We worked with a couple of procedures (the silent 'la, la, la'; the whispered 'ah'; and counting aloud) that encouraged long and relaxed exhalations – which in turn triggered reflexive and automatic inhalations. I explained to Edward that he didn't have to 'do' anything to breathe. When breathing coordination is activated, it's not necessary to muscle the breath; proper breathing is reflexive and involuntary.

Over the course of a year, Edward began to use his body as a feedback system. By changing the habits that were causing his headaches, muscular tension and emotional stress, his pain gradually disappeared. He developed an awareness of himself and a conscious control of his physical and respiratory patterns. Edward became a real believer in the Alexander Technique – which, for him, inspired greater freedom and the benefits of improved health.

BIBLIOGRAPHY

Alexander, F.M. (1995) *A New Method of Respiratory Vocal Re-Education* (1906). Introduction. Articles and Lectures. London: Mouritz.

Stough, C. (1970) *Dr. Breath*. New York: William Morrow and Company.

SECTION 2

Breath and the Mind

JANE BOSTON AND RENA COOK

Western Cartesian-formulated methodologies clearly make a distinction between body and mind as separate entities. By way of a challenge to this, many pedagogical techniques attempt to foster stronger links between breath, the individual and their physical presence. Eastern thought, however, already assumes that breath contributes profoundly to the interconnection of body and mind and aims to make ever more explicit the breath's role in enabling higher states of mindful presence for the performer.

Much of the current dialogue between practitioners falls into this critical territory. Many of those who are most profoundly interested in exploring the embodiment of mind in the body, linking Eastern thought and practice with the West, are currently the most active contemporary bodywork researchers. Taking the position that breath in and of itself is a contributor both to self-knowledge as presence and as a means to communicate with 'truth' to an audience, the authors in the following section each explore the unity of mind/body/breath and its undeniable link to the phenomenon of presence.

Rebecca Cuthbertson-Lane examines the chemistry of breathing function and pursues answers to the question about breath and its relationship to releasing trauma in the body. As a very distinctly interdisciplinary chapter, referring to chemistry, neurology and psychology in her quest for answers, this chapter lays out the strands of the territory and simultaneously makes observations about their synthesis in the process.

Joanna Weir Ouston's account invites readers to make links between psychoanalytic theory and habitual breath patterns. She examines levels of awareness that can be accessed when consciously utilizing the breath as a change agent in relation to performance success and its place in fostering achievement across a range of communicative and physical activities.

Finally, Kristin Linklater poses the idea that an active consciousness of the breathing function will enable the individual to become more available to the audience in ways that are, in her words, 'untrammelled by convention, emotionally and imaginatively daring and... transparent'. In her account, breath enables an advanced state of unmasking the defensive position, thereby genuinely transporting an audience to new levels of imaginative connections.

CHAPTER 5

Breath and the Science of Feeling

Rebecca Cuthbertson-Lane

I am a voice teacher and, as such, work predominantly with actors and actors-in-training. However, my perspective on voicework is not limited to the world of performance; I have, since I first began taking voice classes, developed an acute curiosity with regard to the more holistic/therapeutic aspects of the work that became apparent to me almost immediately. In fact, it was breathwork that ultimately got me hooked on voice. Most of my big 'eureka' moments in the process of working on my own voice occurred during or as a direct result of the practice of breathwork – and deeply profound moments they were. Not just for my voice, but for my whole *being*. I learned first-hand, before I ever looked to make the voice my profession, the power and far-reaching implications of this fundamental physiological process. And partly because it had been so helpful to me, but also because I have witnessed it be so helpful to others in similar ways, I have sought to understand more completely exactly *how* this seemingly simple fuelling mechanism can be so deeply connected to virtually every aspect of who we are and how we live, perceive, interact and communicate – not just on a philosophical or theoretical level, but in actual, measurable, scientific terms.

PART ONE: WHY DO PEOPLE CRY IN VOICE CLASSES?

This question, the original catalyst of my research, arises from a phenomenon that has been experienced by many voice students, witnessed by voice teachers and documented in many voicework texts – namely, the sudden, spontaneous and often uncontrollable release of emotion, most notably in the form of weeping, though it can take other forms as well.[1] Invariably, this phenomenon is attributed to a release of chronic physical tension as a result of relaxation and breathwork and the subsequent liberation of repressed emotions. This explanation, intuitively and in terms of clinical experience, seems correct and among practitioners is never disputed – though the scientific and medical establishments would be likely to take issue with it. It is the *mind*, they argue, not the body, that knows, feels, processes information, initiates responses, remembers and emotes. Experience, of course, teaches us otherwise, so we must break with convention in order to begin to understand this phenomenon and its relevance to our work, either as voice teachers, or as holistic practitioners. This does not mean, however, that we must give up science. New evidence emerges every day that destabilizes the traditional Cartesian mind/body divide and provides support for a holistic, integrated model with endless significance for anyone who works in fields of self-development and health. Because breath is so firmly rooted in both the realms of the body and the mind, it is inevitable that the answer to the question 'why do people cry in voice classes?' is tied to the breath.

Why ask this question?

In the world of voice teachers, there is sometimes a great chasm in the landscape of our understanding of the voice. We are used to dealing with and thinking in terms of, *technique* – the purely physical aspects of healthy, effective voice production that involve muscles, ligaments and cartilage. This is the side of the chasm where many of us are most comfortable. However, we often find that pure technique is prone to fail us; sometimes, certain unhealthy physical habits refuse to shift, or we meet with a student's seemingly inexplicable angry resistance to an exercise – or someone ends up in floods of tears. This is when we must visit the other side of the chasm and acknowledge that there is a very strong *emotional* aspect to our work – one that we simply don't understand very well. The chasm in our knowledge, then, has to do with exactly *how* these two aspects of our work interact and influence one another.

---

1   Since I began my own journey in voice, breath and bodywork, I have met and worked with many holistic health practitioners of various disciplines who assure me that this phenomenon occurs frequently in their treatment rooms in response to all manner of touch and non-touch forms of therapeutic bodywork. As the focus of this book is the power of breath, I will limit my discussion to this aspect of the work; however, most of the information contained here applies to any form of bodywork that involves the application of pressure or the manipulation/transmission of energy.

To a great degree, the rather scary, rather rickety bridge connecting the two has to do with 'trauma'. This is what we, as voice teachers or as practitioners of any and all holistic health paradigms, need to understand better: 'what is trauma?', 'how does trauma work?' and 'what does trauma do to us?' In this process, we come to learn how breathwork provides us with one of the most powerful tools we have to help repair or perhaps even *replace* this bridge with a stronger, more supportive structure.

What do we know already?

In general, the work of voice teachers is to help our students to become aware of and learn to shift, physical tensions that obstruct healthy, effective vocal function. We work from the point of view that, as muscles and joints throughout the body adjust themselves to maintain physical balance, tension held anywhere in the body has a knock-on effect *through* the body and will ultimately affect the breath and the voice, in terms of quality, health and power. We seek, therefore, to release this tension in order to also release the voice and free expression. We know, just as holistic health practitioners know, that chronic tension is both a result and a reflection of one's overall emotional health and that this same chronic tension prevents one from experiencing and responding to the world and other humans freely, spontaneously, generously, healthfully and comfortably. From a purely vocal perspective, we also know that this affects good communication and expressivity and that in order to help students improve these aspects of their lives, we must address unhealthy and inefficient habits of breath and body use.

What is a habit?

A physical habit (distinct, here, from 'addiction') begins with an in-the-moment reaction to a stimulus – often a physical or emotional discomfort or pain that we learn to numb or avoid by assuming a certain shape or affecting a certain behaviour. If the pain or discomfort persists and we continue to assume the physical shape or behaviour that helps us to cope on some level, the behaviour becomes both a self-conditioned behaviour, reinforced through 'muscle memory' *and* an ongoing, in-the-moment reflection of one's relationship with and reaction to the world. In other words, a lot of 'baggage' (or trauma) comes with a habit and it is difficult to address the latter without being confronted with the limiting effects of the former.

Of course, it is certainly possible to train the body to learn a new behaviour – for example, to develop greater flexibility in the ribs in the breathing process. However, without acknowledging that there are *reasons* for the tightness in the ribcage – often, *emotional* reasons – inculcating the new behaviour may always be an uphill battle and may not necessarily create broad-reaching, permanent shifts in the pattern. Working with the voice, therefore, is not simply about breaking someone of bad habits or training them to assume more effective habits. Working with the voice requires us to address and support the *whole* being.

What are the potential benefits?

The benefits of shifting trauma from the body are myriad: people report increased energy, groundedness, vitality, focus, physical freedom and flexibility, among many other benefits, including improvement in overall mental and physical health – all of which are of obvious benefit, whether the beneficiary is an actor-in-training or a patient.

How do I help achieve this?

Although most bodywork paradigms are excellent in terms of freeing the body of tension, stagnant energy and trapped emotion, there is one very simple practice that is of extreme benefit, but which is often overlooked: the breath. Breath and trauma are intimately connected on many levels, as we shall discover. Conscious, sensitive use of breathwork, whether in voice classes or as a part of other bodywork practices, can therefore provide a gentle yet powerful tool in the process of releasing trauma.

PART TWO: TRAUMA STIMULUS AND RESPONSE
What *is* 'trauma'?

This is the first question we must answer if we are to understand the means by which trauma is processed by, held within and, ideally, *released from* the body. According to Cambridge University's online dictionary, trauma is either 'a severe injury, usually caused by a violent attack or an accident', or a 'severe emotional shock and pain caused by an extremely upsetting experience'. What is becoming clear, however, is that it is not simply one or the other of these two possibilities. If it is one, it is simultaneously the other; they are indivisible.

The sources of trauma, generally, can be either low-grade but prolonged or from a singular, high-intensity experience and can be of primarily a physical or an emotional nature – each having a simultaneous reality in the other. An example of a low-grade but prolonged, *physical* source of trauma might be the result of an injury, the on-going pain from which causes one to change one's shape or body use in order to compensate for or avoid the discomfort triggered by the injury. The initial injury itself might be an example of a singular, high-intensity trauma. In either case, there will be a simultaneous emotional response that corresponds in intensity. Similarly, an example of a singular, high-intensity *emotional* trauma might be the su̇ of a loved one, while an example of a low-grade but prolonged trauma might ongoing grief caused by this loss. Again, in either case, the emotional trauma t̪ on, simultaneously, a life in the body, affecting one's shape and body use.

If these are potential *sources* of trauma, the question then becomes one of under-standing how these stimuli are received and processed by the body to produce the individual's responses to the stimulus. These processes are multitudinous and layered and it is impossible to account for them all within the scope of this article. However, we will look at some of the major contributors.

The somatic architecture of trauma: neurological and neuromuscular pathways

Perhaps the most well known trauma-related process initiated by the body is com-monly referred to as the 'fight or flight' response. This complex response involves many systems operating together and virtually instantaneously to help the individ-ual avoid a source of danger. The instant the brain registers a potential threat, the Sympathetic Nervous System (SNS) is activated, triggering a cascade of electrical, neurochemical and hormonal information transmission throughout the body (Siegel 2006, pp. 382–6).

The aspects of the fight or flight response that are most relevant to the analysis of trauma have to do with the effects of stress chemicals and nerve impulses on the re-spiratory, circulatory and muscular systems. These chemical and electrical signals ini-tiate rapid, clavicular breathing, for example, which is important in an actual physical emergency in that it charges the blood and muscle tissue with vital oxygen, but also in that it *dis*charges the excess carbon dioxide that is produced in vigorous activity such as fighting or fleeing. The problem with this process occurs, however, when no immediate *actively* physical response to the perceived threat is required, such as when the individual remains in a heightened state of alertness or emotion over a prolonged period of time. In such a case, this high, rapid breathing pattern is unbeneficial for several reasons (Lewis 1997, p. 54).

One reason is that the carbon dioxide levels in the bloodstream become depleted causing 'respiratory alkalosis'. This condition is advantageous in the event of actual physical trauma in that it has a desensitizing effect on the brain and body, making the whole system less susceptible to pain and that it causes contraction of the blood vessels, which inhibits blood loss. In the uninjured body, however, respiratory alka-losis inhibits blood flow, which in turn reduces oxygenation and detoxification of the tissues and can, furthermore, lead to dizziness, impaired concentration, impaired memory and feelings of disconnection and depersonalization (Saraswati 1999, p. 28). Combined with the stimulating effect that stress chemicals have on the muscular system, respiratory alkalosis can result in intensified contraction of the muscle fibres, owing to the unreleased charge and the retention of toxins in the tissue. To make matters worse, the imbalance in the blood gases can be interpreted as evidence of further danger by the brain, which then triggers the release of more stress chemicals, leaving the individual in a continual, heightened state of tension and arousal (Lewis 1997, pp. 36–7, p. 54).

Regardless of the nature of the stressor, whether physical, psychological or emotional, when the subsequent charge remains unreleased, the combined effects of the fight/flight response result in pockets of dense, rigid, contracted tissue throughout the body, which inevitably affect one's patterns of body use. When this occurs over a prolonged period of time, these patterns become ingrained in the system via two separate but mutually supportive processes. In the first process, the brain *learns* about the new way of being/moving and forges new neural pathways throughout the brain and central nervous system and their neuromuscular connections to support and facilitate the new architecture of the body – as well as dissolving old neural pathways that are now obsolete. This is what we generally understand and refer to as 'muscle memory'.

The second process involves the connective tissue of the body, which includes macro-structures such as ligaments and tendons, but also microstructures such as collagen crystals. This tissue comprises a highly dynamic, plastic system that responds efficiently to patterns of body use, contributing both flexibility and stability. To accomplish this well, the cells and fibres of the connective tissue align themselves along the lines of tension in the body – that is, the structure of the system and its individual components is determined by the tensional stressors/usage patterns to which it is subjected. In practice, this means that when an individual changes his/her pattern of body use over an extended period of time, the connective tissue responds by changing its own shape in order to maintain the overall balance and harmony of the body. Ultimately, then, the patterns of body use become manifested as *form* – not just as a matter of habit, but as an inherent aspect of one's physical structure. This can be seen as a kind of somatic memory, as the original trauma is stored in the body as a physical *shape* (Oschman 2003b, p. 276).

What role do emotions play in this process?

In a life-or-death situation (or one that is perceived, psychologically, with a similar gravity), emotions are extravagant and potentially deadly indulgences, so the body makes sure to push them down, enabling it to focus on saving itself. The system is set up to react *now* and feel later, when the individual has the luxury of time and safety to process these strong emotions. However, if prolonged stress or re-current trauma leave the body in a continual state of tension, it is extremely difficult to get to the 'feel' part, let alone to express it. The unreleased emotions then exacerbate the problem, adding ever-deepening layers of tension, inhibition and repression.

PART THREE: SOMATIC MEMORY, SOMATIC THERAPY AND BREATH
Philosophy meets science

Various therapeutic paradigms have evolved over the past century that have acknowledged the body's role in the processing and storage of trauma and traumatic memory and have therefore used the body as the primary focus of treatment. Wilhelm Reich was the first notable 'somatic therapist' (and certainly one of the most influential, considering the number of his 'disciples' who have developed their own therapeutic paradigms), but others, such as Stanley Keleman, have made significant contributions to this new branch of healing theory. Regardless of the practitioner or the name they give to their brand of therapy, they all seem to hold three important concepts as fundamental: 1) the body and mind are indivisible, 2) the traumas to which an individual is subjected are stored in the body as form (through tension) and 3) the breath is a crucial aspect of both repressing and *releasing* trauma. Keleman effectively summarizes this breath connection when he notes:

> (a)n individual who will not fully inhale will not fully inspire himself, accept into himself the influx of his surround. An individual who inhibits exhaling will not fully commit himself, give himself trustingly to his surround. An individual who will not fully breathe restricts his individuality. (1981, p.154)

Freeing the breath is therefore of fundamental importance in the process of freeing the whole of the person from their traumatic histories – physically, psychologically and emotionally.

It may be tempting to see these somatic therapy models as merely philosophical or metaphorical. There is, however, a significant (and rapidly growing), scientific body of evidence to support these ideas and show them to be much closer to reality than the established paradigms of western medicine and science have been prepared to acknowledge. In his two books, *Energy Medicine: The Scientific Basis* and *Energy Medicine in Therapeutics and Human Performance*, Dr James Oschman compiles a tremendous amount of data derived from hundreds of scientific studies and presents a cogent, cohesive argument for the existence and functioning of a unifying energy system in the body that is responsible for both the holding and the releasing of tension and trauma.

The fundamental premise underlying Oschman's work is that body, mind, emotions and intellect exist as *one* cohesive whole and that anything that occurs in one aspect of the whole directly affects every other aspect of the whole. In his model, any localised stimulus is *instantaneously* processed as information throughout the being and thus triggers many of the biological processes that ultimately serve to keep the individual in harmony and balance within itself. This essential 'one-ness' of the self is attributable, Oschman's research shows, through a system he calls 'the living matrix'.

'The living matrix' concept holds that the body consists of multitudinous cells embedded in and connected to an uninterrupted, intricate network of extra-cellular connective tissue made up primarily of collagen crystals (Oschman 2003a, p. 47). This matrix is 'a continuous and dynamic "supra-molecular" web-work, extending into every nook and cranny of the body'. Thus, when you touch a human body, you are touching a continuously inter-connected system where 'effects on one part of the system can and do spread to others' (2003a, p. 48). Sensory, motor and regulatory information from any part of the body is available to the entire system instantaneously.

This interconnectivity is possible in Oschman's model because is it predicated on the idea that the body's processes are not only bio-electrical and bio-magnetic in nature (as in established paradigms), they are also *bio-electronic*. Oschman asserts that the collagenous liquid-crystal protein structures that comprise the matrix serve as *semi-conductors* (2003b, pp. 270-1) that are able 'to conduct, process *and store* energy and information of various kinds', in much the same way that modern electronic and computer systems do (2003b, p. 90). This system makes it possible for instantaneous processing and flow of information throughout the body, allowing the body to fine-tune all of its regulatory functions and maintain its balance and health.

Another key factor contributing to the body's fundamental inter-connectedness is what Oschman refers to as 'tensegrity'[2]. A tensegrity system is a stable yet dynamic system, 'characterised by a continuous tensional network (tendons) connected by a discontinuous set of compressive elements (struts)' that 'interacts efficiently and resiliently with forces acting on it' (2003a, p. 153). According to Oschman, the entire body is comprised of various micro- and macro-cosmic tensegrity systems, from the

---

2   From 'tensional integrity' (Oschman 2003:66), an architectural concept developed by R. Buckminster Fuller, and the principle underlying flexible but stable structures such as tents and geodesic domes.

body as a whole to the DNA itself (2003a, p. 63–7). In terms of the holistic nature of the system then, tensegrity works *mechanically* – if you move or change even just one aspect of a tensegral system, the entire system shifts to accommodate it – but also *energetically*. Oschman points out that if you pluck or strike one of the tendons or jar one of the struts of a tensegrity model, the *entire* network will vibrate (2003a, p. 66). The key link between the energetic and mechanical functions that unify the entire bodily system, then, is vibration.

Functionally, this is an ideal working system. All parts of the body are in continual vibrational contact with all other parts of the body and can adjust to the slightest imbalance immediately in order to safeguard the whole. The only problem with it surfaces when prolonged emotional or physical trauma puts higher than average stress on the system. Tissues that have become rigid, contracted and dense through the accumulated effects of trauma effectively break the continuum of vibratory information and energy flow. Oschman explains that under these circumstances,

> Connective tissue fibres bunch up, forming dense regions at the ends of tendons and ligaments where they attach to bones. This 'kinking' of the collagen bundles shortens the tendon or ligament, tenses the muscles and strains joints. Lack of motion and poor circulation to these dense regions leads to dehydration and shrinking of the ground substance.[3] Cells become energetically isolated from the living matrix. (2003a, p. 171)

It is then difficult for the body to heal or re-balance itself because there is no way of communicating effectively, through the usual vibrational channels, with the affected tissue.

As a means of overcoming this block in the 'circuitry', Oschman proposes any of several 'bodywork' paradigms (a list which is incomplete without breathwork), as they serve to re-integrate the compromised tissue into the energetic matrix through the effects of *pressure*. The significant improvement in the plasticity of tissue subjected to pressure is attributable to the fact that when this sort of force/energy is applied to colloidal gel, it quickly turns to 'sol', a more liquid, though still viscous, form of the substance. The tissue is thus re-hydrated, re-aligned and re-connected to the vibratory energy/information flow of the matrix (Oschman 2003a, pp. 170-1). It is for this reason that breathwork must necessarily be included in Oschman's list of useful bodywork paradigms; the pressure forces involved in the full expansion and contraction activities of the diaphragm and the ribs contribute significantly to the release and realignment of tissues throughout the entire torso.

---

3   Colloidal gel is 'the universal internal environment' surrounding all tissue cells and the collagen fibres of the living matrix. (2003:169).

Oschman's work in these two texts goes on to explore other aspects of the body/breath/emotion equation that are directly relevant to understanding the complex processes at work in the storage of trauma within the body and the methods through which it is most effectively released – most of which are too complicated to explore within the scope of this article. One important aspect of the body/breath/emotion equation that Oschman does not address, however, is what emotion actually *is*. For this, we turn to Candace Pert, a neuroscientist who has made significant contributions to her field, particularly with regard to advancing our understanding of emotion and the *neurochemical* processes that account for our experience of them.

Neurochemistry: another scientific perspective

As we come to terms with the concept of the body being, essentially, a medium for the transmission, processing and storage of various forms of energy/vibration at varying frequencies (and the effects these vibrations have on the body), we learn that what is at the heart of all this energy flow is *information*. For Pert, emotions are simply another aspect of the body's information exchange processes and thus are able to flow, influence behaviour and sensation, *or be stored* – such as in the case of repressed emotions and trauma.

We have established that the sensation of unpleasant emotion can cause a person to adopt unhealthy physical habits as coping mechanisms and thereby cause damage to the tissues involved and to the whole system, ultimately. However, it is not yet clear how releasing this tissue subsequently releases the emotion. Pert offers an explanation in the form of biochemicals: 'opiate receptors', 'ligands' and 'neuropeptides'. In essence, Dr Pert has determined that emotions have a *chemical* structure and, at the molecular level, specific vibrational patterns that allow them to interact with and affect the various structures of the body. 'Neuropeptide' molecules are, she says, the 'molecules of emotion' named in the title of her book. A form of 'ligand'[4], neuropeptides react exclusively with 'opiate receptors' located in cells throughout the brain as well as throughout the entire body (Pert 1997, p. 72).

The fact that these neuropeptides and their receptors are located in the brain *and* in the body has led Pert to speculate that the classic Cartesian division between mind and body mentioned earlier can no longer be so vehemently upheld within the scientific community (1997, p. 188). She proposes that they are, in fact, *one thing* – leading her to adopt the term 'bodymind' when referring to the complex processes

---

4   A ligland is any migatory molecule in the body that binds with specific 'receptor' molecules embedded on the surface of every cell of the body and that thus provides the cell with information regarding the regulation of it's internal mechanisms.

that affect the entire organism at once, particularly those that are caused by emotion (1997, p. 187).

In essence, according to Pert, what we experience as emotion is simply the effects wrought by the 'free flow of information carried by the bio-chemicals of emotion, the neuropeptides and their receptors' (1997, p. 276). With regard to how this 'free flow' becomes staunched and how emotions and other forms of memory are stored in the tissue of the entire body, Pert explains that when receptors are flooded with a particular neuropeptide (for example, endorphins, an endogenous chemical generally associated with 'feel-good' states), they stimulate a specific electrical impulse within the cell membrane that both penetrates into the cell – instructing it with regard to what processes to initiate – and triggers a specific neuronal circuit to be activated in the nervous system. When the same, precise neuronal pathways are activated again and again, the thoughts/experiences they codify are more likely to become a permanent part of the psyche – as memory. Therefore, 'the decision about what becomes a thought rising to consciousness and what remains an undigested thought pattern buried at a deeper level of the body is mediated by the receptors and this includes *emotional* memory (1997, p. 143).

Another important aspect of Pert's explanation of emotional memory has to do with the means by which the neuropeptides and their receptors find one another and subsequently bind together – a process that is *vibratory* in nature. Pert describes the process as being like 'two voices – ligand and receptor – striking the same note' (1997, p. 24), an occurrence which essentially amounts to an exchange of information. The process is both chemical and energetic/vibrational in nature and requires, therefore, healthy, vibrant, hydrated, energetically-conductive tissue, connected to the 'living matrix' to serve as the medium for the information flow that will trigger the physiological changes in the body that we experience as emotion.

If emotions are triggered – that is, if the neuropeptides linked with that emotional state are released into the blood stream and throughout the ground substance – and then subsequently *suppressed* through tension, the neuropeptides and receptors will be unable to find one another. The chemicals will be present in the tissue, but until they are free to flow and diffuse efficiently through the cellular environment, they will be simply stuck and never make contact with their receptors. Thus, no information will be transmitted, no physiological changes in the body will be initiated and no 'feelings' will be perceived by the conscious mind.

With the conscious application of body and breathwork activities, however, this tissue is re-integrated into the network, vibrational energy flow is facilitated and emotion-chemical molecules are released. At this point, they either become attached to new receptors and, thus, experienced as an emotion (including, potentially but not inevitably, the memory that triggered it) or are processed as toxins and eliminated from the body via the breath (often as a sigh or breathy shudder, but sometimes as laughter or sobbing), tears, skin or excretory systems. In either case, the individual is freer of both physical tension and the suppressed emotion that prompted it.

PART FOUR: DEEPER CONNECTIONS TO BREATHWORK
Breathing and speaking 'from the gut'

While the above material goes a certain distance toward explaining how breath-work is beneficial in a general, tension-releasing/emotional-flow kind of way, voice teachers have a particular understanding, however intuitive or theoretical its base, of the special link that exists between the breath, the emotions and 'the gut'. Voice teachers regularly encourage students to 'connect with and speak from the centre' or 'the core' in a reference that is linked to, but not entirely the same as, using one's abdominal support. What we mean by this is that we want students to connect with their deepest emotional resources and to truly commit to expressing what they find there. Instinctively, we know that one may only accomplish this by engaging and accessing the special energies available in 'the gut'. However, this phenomenon is not simply a metaphorical or philosophical concept; it has a basis in physiology and is connected with the same neurological, neurochemical and energetic systems Pert and Oschman discuss. In fact, a relatively new field of scientific inquiry, called 'neuro-gastroenterology', has evolved to explore what can be referred to as 'the brain in the gut', otherwise known as the 'Enteric Nervous System' (ENS).

The ENS is comprised of tissue lining the oesophagus, stomach, large and small intestines and the colon (Gershon 1998, p. 113). According to researchers, this 'brain-like' system has more than one hundred million nerve cells in the small intestine alone, (a number roughly equal to the number of nerve cells in the spinal cord) and more *total* nerve cells than 'the entire remainder of our peripheral nervous system'. In fact, the brain and the ENS are each formed in the embryo out of the same clump of tissue (called the 'neural crest'), which divides early in the development of the fetus and is only later re-connected via a cable called the 'vagus nerve' (Gershon 1998, pp. 241-4). The vagus is a cranial nerve of the parasympathetic nervous system that 'in-nervates the entire gut from the oesophagus all the way down to the middle of the colon' (1998, p. 19).

The ENS is also 'a vast chemical warehouse within which is represented every one of the classes of neurotransmitter found in the brain' (Gershon 1998, p. xiii). Given the fact that the 'entire lining of the intestines, from the oesophagus through the large intestine and including each of the seven sphincters, is lined with cells...

that contain neuropeptides and receptors' (Pert 1997, p. 188) it is, indeed, very much like a second brain in that it is able to send and receive neurochemical impulses, respond to emotions and record experiences to be stored as memory. It is these complex neural and neurochemical connections, then, that make it possible for us to have what many refer to as 'gut feelings'. However, the brain-like qualities of the ENS also make this area of the body a great potential storehouse for trauma.

What is the connection between the ENS and breathwork?

The ENS communicates with the various other branches of the nervous system through neural connections in the spine, but also through the vagus nerve. As mentioned above, the vagus nerve is one of the major structures of the PNS, the branch of the ANS responsible for *counteracting* the effects of stimulation to the SNS (i.e. the 'fight or flight' response); its role is to help soothe, calm and balance the body. The vagus nerve emerges from the brainstem and descends downward through the body, penetrating the diaphragm to connect with the ENS. Along the way, it supplies motor parasympathetic nerve fibres to all the organs except the adrenal glands from the neck down to the colon and also controls a few skeletal muscles, such as the pharyngeal constrictors and the muscles of the larynx required for voice production.

In essence, once the SNS initiates its fight or flight response, dilating the bronchial passages and arresting peristaltic activity in the bowel, etc., the PNS – via the motor neurons of the vagus nerve – goes to work to bring harmony back to the system; it narrows the air passages to prevent over-breathing, calms the heart rate and initiates the peristaltic activities that are required for such things as proper digestion and elimination. However, when the vagus nerve is *over*-stimulated, as occurs when it is working hard to balance a prolonged or frequently recurring stress response, it can cause the throat to tighten (restricting breath) and the bowel to over-react, potentially leading to nausea, 'butterflies' and other unpleasant nervous digestive responses (Gershon 1998, p. 105).

Conscious breathing, however, can help to normalize all of these hyperactive systems and processes and it is able to accomplish this via various mechanisms. First, the diaphragm makes active contact with the vagus, repeatedly stroking and stimulating the sensory neurons of the PNS, thus transmitting a message of calm and harmony that spreads throughout the CNS (Sapolsky 2004, p. 38). Furthermore, conscious breathing regulates and balances the blood gases, preventing the destructive cycle caused respiratory alkalosis discussed earlier. Together, these effects work to counteract the cumulative damage wrought by an over-stimulated SNS; they help to release some of the chemical charge in the muscle tissue and allow the body to re-absorb or eliminate the over-abundant hormones and neurotransmitters associated with the stress response, thus reducing the level of tension and contraction in the muscle tissue. The body can then re-harmonize its functions and structural imbalances. When patterns and habits ingrained through *chronic* SNS over-stimulation (ongoing stress and trauma) emerge, however, conscious breathing can work in deeper, more complex ways to help free the body of both the tensions *and* the trauma, as we shall see as we explore further.

PART FIVE: SO... *WHY* DO PEOPLE CRY IN VOICE CLASSES?

Having laid this groundwork, we now return to the original question. Breathwork, it seems, is able to work on many levels to serve in the process of healing damaged or rigid tissue, connecting with suppressed emotions and providing the means through which they can be released from the body. Mechanically, the pressure force exerted on the tissues directly affected by the expansion of the lungs and the descent of the diaphragm during inspiration initiates the gel-to-sol mechanism that allows release and re-alignment of contracted collagen crystals, thus freeing and re-invigorating dense, rigid muscles, tendons, etc., throughout the entire torso. Energetically, this same pressure force allows vibrations to flow more freely through the entire body, helping to release rigid tissue in areas not directly touched by the mechanical pulse of the breath. Chemically, the emotional energy encapsulated in the neuropeptides and freed in the process of unlocking the dense tissue is then provided with a current of energy on which to move – partly on the strength of the vibrations themselves and partly via the mechanical waves initiated by the expansion/contraction of the breathing rhythm. The emotion is no longer trapped; it is free to flow, to be felt, experienced, connected with and *expressed*.

The significance of this model is strengthened when one considers the direct contact the breathing rhythm, with all its multi-faceted effects, has with the ENS, which is an area particularly susceptible to the detrimental effects of stress, trauma and repressed emotions. Its unique physiological and neurological aspects combine to create a system of profound sensitivity on an emotional level. It is easy to see, then, why one might habitually arrest one's breathing in order to block oneself off from an experience of such potential turmoil. Good breathing requires the release of muscles intimately connected with this tissue – the diaphragm, the abdominals and the deep support muscles of the spine – not to mention the softening of the organs and other tissues of the lower torso. When these tissues are soft and flexible, there can be no disconnection from the emotions so often held there. The pressure force involved in the descension of the diaphragm encourages ongoing release of the tissues in the gut, allowing them to stay connected, energetically, to the 'living matrix' and thus, promoting the free-flow of information chemicals through this highly sensitive 'second brain'. It then becomes impossible to ignore or otherwise repress one's deepest feelings and so, after a certain amount of body and breath work, people may end up experiencing a spontaneous release of long-held emotions.

What are the potential implications of this work, psychologically?

The scenario outlined above is potentially frightening and overwhelming, particularly if the repressed trauma is exceptionally painful; however, it is often the case, in terms of processing the trauma, that simply *breathing through* the release is enough. Swami Ambikananda Saraswati, a Yogini and breathing expert, maintains that Yoga, for example,

> does not require the full recall of any of the emotions that may have provoked a life-long habit of tension. To the Yogi, the tightened, tense muscle is the body's way of remembering the trauma and restoring that muscle to its resting length *is* the complete release. (Saraswati 1999, p. 42)

She is clear throughout her text that good breathing is an integral part of this process. To some degree, then, it may be said that simply doing the work – gently, gradually and with conscious attunement to good (i.e. *free, abdominal*) breathing practice – *is* the process of healing from and releasing traumas. Regardless of the bodywork paradigm in which one works, therefore, learning to breathe more effectively and more healthfully – and then teaching this to one's clients/patients/students can only support and, indeed, magnify the good work that is already occurring. Just be sure to keep a box of tissues handy.

AN EPILOGUE FOR VOICE TEACHERS
What are the further implications of this work for an actor, or someone who works with actors?

The concepts outlined above have tremendous significance for an actor, since any 'athletic, artistic and intellectual performance is enhanced when all of the body's communication channels are open and balanced' (Oschman 2003, p. 90). As voice teachers, we know that accessing the power inherent in emotionally challenging texts requires that the actor be particularly free and available, both physically and vocally. Breathing freely is thus important to an actor in that it provides a direct connection between the physical, vocal and *emotional* aspects of performance and that it allows him/her to be more 'in the moment'. As we discovered earlier, many of the effects of SNS stimulation have a de-sensitizing effect on the body, in order to allow the organism to continue to function despite potential pain and trauma in the struggle for survival. These anaesthetizing and depersonalizing effects are, by design, a barrier to emotional connection and expressivity both within and outside of the acting process. The deliberate activation of the PNS (via contact with the vagus nerve) and the re-stabilization of the blood gases that occur through the process of conscious breathing allow us to reconnect with the world around us. For the actor, this means being fully 'present' – reacting spontaneously and without inhibition to impulses that are now free to arise.

As voice teachers, we are and must be concerned with technique. It is without doubt the cornerstone of our teaching. However, when confronted with seemingly unshiftable habits, technique can only take us a certain distance in a certain, specific direction. The voice cannot be treated as a mechanism that simply needs the odd adjustment to function more effectively. As a reflection of a person's whole being, the voice must be treated holistically, i.e. in order to access the full spectrum of a person's physical/vocal/emotional potential, one must *address* the full spectrum of the person's physical/vocal/emotional challenges. Understanding the means by which trauma of any sort becomes integrated into the whole of the body and self, and one of the key mechanisms through which it is released, may go a long way to relieving the fear and anxiety that both practitioners and students may feel in those moments when a seemingly simple voice or breathing exercise triggers something profoundly personal in someone vulnerable. Trusting that it is a healthy, often necessary, process can allow everyone involved to breathe a little more easily.

BIBLIOGRAPHY

Gershon, M. (1998) *The Second Brain*. New York: Harper Collins.

Keleman, S. (1981) *Your Body Speaks Its Mind*. Berkeley (CA): Center Press.

Lewis, D. (1997) *The Tao of Natural Breathing*. San Francisco: Mountain Wind.

Oschman, J. (2003a) *Energy Medicine: The Scientific Basis*. London: Churchill Livingstone.

Oschman, J. (2003b) *Energy Medicine in Therapeutics and Human Performance*. London: Butterworth Heinemann.

Pert, C. (1997) *Molecules of Emotion*. London: Simon and Schuster.

Sapolsky, R. (2004) *Why Zebras Don't Get Ulcers*, 3rd ed. New York: Owl Books.

Siegel, A. (2006) *Essential Neuroscience*, revised 1st ed. Baltimore: Lippincott, Williams and Wilkins.

Saraswati, Swami A. (1999) *Principles of Breathwork*. London: Thorson's.

CHAPTER 6

The Breathing Mind, the Feeling Voice

Exploring the connection between breath, voice and emotion

JOANNA WEIR OUSTON

> When you meditate, remember your breath:
> Thanks to it, man has come alive.
>
> Fr. Seraphion of Mount Athos

Ancient peoples often referred to breath as the life force, and certainly breathing is one of the most primary and critical bodily functions. Breath is so essential to life that we can only survive minutes without it, whereas we can go several days without water and weeks without food. Yet, respiration is one of the most underestimated of bodily functions. Most of the time we aren't consciously aware of breathing so we take it for granted that we are performing this function well.

While it would be widely agreed that breathing is a vital physical function which fuels the body, few people would think of it as having any direct impact on the mind or emotional life. Breath can express emotion or state of mind (such as fear, joy, arousal, anxiety or relief) and breath also can be used to create or suppress emotion. Although we regard breathing as being essential to life, we seldom realize the impact it can have on quality of life.

In fact, the way in which we breathe has profound psycho-physical ramifications on every aspect of our lives, from health and emotional outlook, to confidence levels, ability to communicate and the way in which we perform under pressure. Consequently, breath lies at the very heart of an individual's sense of self and at the core of every aspect of daily life. Breath is also the life force of a performance, be it on the stage, in the boardroom, classroom, pulpit, courtroom or any other type of real-life 'stage'. The way in which one breathes – centred or shallow – directly affects one's presence and relationship with the world.

This chapter will explore some of the ways in which habitual breath patterns and vocal usage can affect an individual's psychology and will investigate the influence breath, voice and psychology have on peak performance. An examination of the role the mind plays in voice training and peak performance will also chart some of the contextual complexity within which voice training operates. By its very nature, voice training is attempting to achieve profound psycho-physical change. This requires the re-programming of deep-seated defensive or habitual unconscious neuromuscular responses, all of which are intrinsically linked to the breath pattern. Frequently this change engenders a conscious or unconscious re-alignment of self-image and habitual communication behaviours. Breath is such a powerful restorative force within us that, whether we wish to acknowledge it or not, voice training is ultimately physically and psychologically therapeutic, though it is not psychotherapy.

THE EMOTIONAL BODY-BRAIN

The body plays a pivotal role in our emotional state and our very sense of self. It can even broaden or limit our personal horizons, contributing to our fundamental world-view. Life experience is a very major influence that can shape the way in which we breathe, use our voices, hold ourselves physically, cope with stress and crisis. Breath and alignment lie at the core of the ability to cope. But before we can examine this in more detail we need to understand the symbiotic relationship between the brain, the body and emotions (see Chapter 5 by Rebecca Cuthbertson-Lane).

The direct link between the emotions and the vocal musculature is of major significance. In voice work we are creating at times dramatic changes in the breath, the vocal tract, even in the musculature of the face. We are also working with the alignment of the spine, the head-neck-shoulder relationship, release of tension in the limbs, release of the abdominal and pelvic areas and so on. Consequently, it is not surprising that voice work sometimes elicits emotional responses such as tears, laughter or dizziness. Although many people would probably just report an increased feeling of well-being and resonance from voice work, some experience profound changes to their neural structures. For example, Melanie, a 30-year-old librarian who had very shallow, clavicular breathing, a light breathy voice and under-muscularized articulators, a change in breathing was joyfully cathartic. Whenever she began to engage her breath more deeply – even on the gentlest 'ff' or 'huh' – she laughed uncontrollably, which was excellent because the act of belly laughing engaged her breath even more deeply. It took some time before her breathing could drop without this massive response of sheer, uncontrollable delight, but when it did a beautifully resonant voice and clearer speech began to emerge and importantly, so did a new-found confidence.

In contrast, John, a 45-year-old actor, was surprised when he found tears rolling down his face as he released tension in his tongue root and for Edward, a 50-year-old businessman, it was the release of the jaw together with a marked increase in resonance that brought a simultaneous mixture of tears and exhilaration. On the other hand, Amy, a 22-year-old student who habitually used a very light breathy voice, felt dizzy whenever she tapped a lovely, bright resonance and accessed clear high notes. It wasn't until her body-mind became re-accustomed to the sensation of head resonance that it became natural for her to use that vocal quality again.

In all of these cases, voice and breath work created an emotional response because of the direct link between the vocal apparatus and the emotional centres in the brain. This raises two important questions:

1. Where do the tensions which could give rise to the release of emotions during voice work originate?

2. What causes vocal tension in the first place?

Putting injury, illness and congenital conditions aside, I would suggest there are four main factors which are involved in the development of vocal tension:

1. the process of socialization (in terms of acceptable social behaviour and also gender identity)

2. accent and language

3. muscular tension created by emotional reactions to life experiences

4. the need for rapport, both with family and peer group.

Healthy babies are born with beautifully centred, effective breathing patterns and free, connected voices about which they have no inhibitions or preconceptions. When it comes to crying, this free utilization of the voice may be resolved as quickly as possible by understanding, loving parents who stay calm and nurture the infant back to relaxation. Alternatively, the infant's crying may be ignored for a time, for various reasons, and its distress may have an effect on the baby's tension levels. Therefore, even at this early stage of life we see the potential for the development of tensions in the breathing mechanism and the vocal apparatus.

Fast-forward 18 months to four years and the child is undergoing very rapid socialization. His enthusiastic exploration of his upper registers may be fine at home but could become embarrassing for the parents if they are in a public place. The child is also rapidly learning the types of behaviour that are rewarded or frowned upon and is developing a sense of his or her gender, including gender based voice qualities that are – at this stage – highly influenced by the parents. These unconsciously observed voice qualities may form the habitual muscular 'imprint' of the child's vocal tract for the rest of his life.

It is not uncommon for vocal tensions – and their resultant vocal qualities – to run in families. The hyper-nasality of the mother and daughter, or the tight, throaty sound of the father and son are seldom due to familial idiosyncratic physiology of the vocal tract. If that were the case, voice training would make little fundamental difference. Consequently, there is a strong possibility that mimicry of the parent's vocal setting by the child may create or contribute to vocal tension. Vocal mimicry stems from the need for rapport and a natural inclination towards hero worship, which results in the unconscious copying and adoption of the tensions of the primary role models, whose tensions may, in turn, have also been copied.

As the child grows older the peer group becomes the dominant influence. Consequently, the speech and vocal qualities of the alpha members of the group (and their vocal tensions) may become the dominating influence. So a teenage girl may develop a similar nasal vocal quality to that of her best friend, or a group of teenage boys in good rapport may all slouch, shallow breathe, glottalize and under-articulate their speech.

Importantly, these adopted tensions will have an emotional affect. One cannot shallow breathe, or tighten the throat, or slump in the upper chest without it in some way affecting one's emotional state or life. So it may be that some of our students are carrying around other people's emotional baggage (perhaps several generations old) as well as their own.

Consequently, when we embark on the process of freeing the voice we are working at an extremely profound level within the human organism. The way in which an individual engages his voice and breath is inextricably linked to his identity and the emotional landscape he has constructed in response to his life experiences. When a voice teacher encourages the making of even small changes in areas such as alignment and breath, tension in the root of the tongue, jaw or neck, the pharynx or the habitual setting of the musculature of the face, he or she is having a direct, physiological impact on the student's emotional and psychological life.

When we work with a young woman who habitually uses a 'little girl' voice and help her discover a more richly resonant and womanly tone with deeper harmonics, we are giving her more than just access to a fuller sound and the means by which to create a more effective sound wave. We are providing her with an experience that can change her emotional relationship with the world. The sound may surprise her and she may love it, but she is unlikely to use it in real life until she owns the different feeling of presence and power it gives her.

A student's fear of being less acceptable to his family or peer group and his emotional dependence on their positive feedback also play a key role here. This is very obvious in the area of dialect. Student actors who negatively perceive clear speech or a more standardized accent (e.g. Received Pronunciation) as sounding 'posh' will have more difficulty learning and using it accurately and naturally than those who simply see it as an important tool. Often students confuse speaking clearly with speaking in RP (i.e. 'posh'), so while enunciating their ds, ts, ls and ngs in a voice class is acceptable, asking them to incorporate more muscularity into their daily speech can give rise to heartfelt emotions about the fear of being rejected or belittled by the peer group or family for trying to sound 'different' and 'superior'.

The speech/accent issue is, however, one that is 'above board' and therefore easier to discuss. The vocal quality issue is subtler, consequently students can be in denial about the shift and why it only seems to take place with the help of the voice teacher. The young female student may experience an incredibly resonant voice in exercises, yet when she speaks about her experience it will frequently be with her habitual little girl voice until she is prepared to make an emotional shift with regard to her identity, self image and the way in which she relates to others. Again, pressure from others – real or perceived – is an important factor and I will illustrate this with a real life example.

Rajiv was in his early 40s and spoke with a very high pitched, rather feeble voice. Over the telephone it was difficult to ascertain his gender and the indirect, unsupported quality of his vocal tone would not inspire confidence in others regarding his level of professionalism and, most probably, his mental acuity. Yet, he was physically strong, had a wide neck and large ribcage and was very masculine. He was an intelligent, highly capable and skilled IT specialist who had a rosy future with his employing company. His manager suggested to him that he have some voice training because, for further promotion, his speech needed to be 'clearer'. It was immediately obvious, however, that the real problem was the voice and not the speech. His actual articulation was reasonably clear but his vocal quality was muffled and robbed him of presence and gravitas.

During the very first session Rajiv managed to tap a beautiful, deep, velvety voice. His initial response to the new found resonance was one of disbelief and 'But that's not my voice!' 'Then whose is it?' I asked, 'As it's certainly not mine!' At which point he laughed and began to own what was going on. The change was so dramatic that I felt compelled to counsel him about speaking in this, his true voice, to family and friends who were only used to the very strangled and unsupported voice he habitually used. He thought it would be fine – that there would be no shock for family and that he could easily incorporate it into his daily life. At the second session, although he arrived using his habitually high, tight voice, he managed to tap a deeper resonance more quickly than at the first session and found even greater richness and vocal charisma. He seemed to enjoy the resonance and depth of his voice and his progress was astoundingly good. He left the second session speaking confidently with the newfound resonance.

When he arrived for his third session he had once more reverted to the higher tonal quality. He told me his employer was disappointed because there was no difference in his voice. Although this was not overly surprising given we only had two one-hour sessions, I had expected to hear more evidence of change because of his rapid progress and apparent ownership of the richer resonance. I asked him what happened between our sessions: what sort of practice he was doing and how he was using his voice. He laughed and said that as he arrived home after the voice session his wife would call out to him: 'Just don't bring that voice into the house!' Although I had counselled about introducing his wife to the change in his voice and warned him that she may initially feel somewhat threatened by it, he unfortunately dismissed it as a potential problem. In the end, his everyday speaking voice did become more resonant but development was more gradual because of his wife's emotional responses rather than his own. Consequently, it is vital not to underestimate the pressure which the need for rapport with the family and peer group exerts on vocal identity and usage, and ultimately, on personal power.

THE BODY-MIND-BREATH RELATIONSHIP

Physical alignment has a direct impact on breath and also profoundly affects an individual's relationship with the world: for example, a slumped upper torso withdraws a person's energy and only allows for the engagement of a shallow breath. These have a detrimental affect on core performance factors such as confidence, vocal resonance and gravitas. The breath-body-mind relationship is so powerful that actors use it to create the emotional life of the characters they are playing. Even minor adjustments in body and breath patterns can have a surprisingly powerful influence on mind-set, self-image and communication.

When an actor needs to play a shy, withdrawn, unassuming character he will naturally adopt a cluster of 'flight pattern' physical and vocal behaviours. These may include a slumped torso, raised shoulders, staccato tempo, shallow breath, retracting musculature (so that the body takes up less space), indirect eye contact and a light, uncertain voice – in short, physical and vocal behaviours which withdraw from the communication space and are associated with a lack of confidence. In fact, simply inhabiting the body language of shyness will result in shallow breath and a light, uncertain voice.

Finding the body patterns (which will, in turn, create the breath and vocal patterns) of an emotional state triggers a deep-seated muscle memory which activates the emotional state or mind-set associated with those body-breath-voice patterns. For example, when playing a depressed character, the actor will engage his musculature in a very different way to that of a buoyant, happy, confident character. The actor knows he is only acting, but the feelings and mind-set generated by muscle memory are very real and may make him even tremble or cry. Such is the power of muscle memory and that profound neurological link between the emotions and the body.

The very nature of voice work involves adjustments in alignment, breathing, resonance, physical tension and vocal identity. Consequently, when a voice teacher works with a student, he or she is making adjustments to muscles which may have a direct impact on the student's emotional landscape. In fact, the teacher is subliminally altering the student's emotional relationship with the world – possibly from one of fear, to confidence and ease. So when we work with someone's breath we are not just changing the mechanics of breathing, spine alignment or vocal quality, we are actually changing his or her life in some way. The combined force of habitual breathing patterns, physical alignment and vocal usage tie in so intimately with fundamental elements of identity that all work on voice and breath has profound emotional and psychological implications.

The close connection the body and vocal tract have with the emotional centres of the brain is a major determining factor both on mind-set and the ability to perform well under pressure. Performance anxiety and breath lie at the heart of our ability to think positively and control our nerves. This profound inter-relationship between the mind, breath and performance continually affects our daily lives, both through self-image and self esteem, as well as the ability to handle pressure.

It is exceedingly clear that changing the breath pattern can change an individual's emotional state. In other words, breath pattern can both reflect and create the way a person feels. This phenomenon is so potent it is employed in psychotherapy as an aid in the management of stress and phobias.

BREATH AND PEAK PERFORMANCE

The sporting world has long been investigating the psychology of success. Every professional coach knows that getting sports people psychologically 'in the zone' is as important as ensuring they are physically in top form. The body-mind relationship is crucial to achieving peak performance and the centred breath lies at the core of this relationship. Performance anxiety can inspire or debilitate sportsmen, actors and business people alike. At its extreme, it manifests itself in the actor as stage fright, whereas in its more minor incarnation it simply renders a performance less successful. Yet, ironically, some performance anxiety is necessary. Every performer knows that without a frisson of nerves there is frequently a danger of mediocrity. The answer to this conundrum lies in finding the right balance between adrenalin and relaxation. In other words, adrenalin harnessed by a centred breath pattern helps create ease, focus and clarity of mind (see Chapter 12 by Rena Cook).

At the heart of this balance is the fight-or-flight instinct. The efficacy with which a performer handles this directly determines levels of anxiety, vocal resonance, charisma and performance success. Breath provides a direct route for accessing and channelling this very powerful instinct.

If a performer's breath isn't sufficiently centred, the unconscious mind simply will not believe the positive success messages and visualizations the performer is consciously trying hang onto. Furthermore, the unconscious mind will actively undermine the conscious mind's attempts at getting into the right, confident mind-set. This is because the shallow breathing pattern and physical tension created by a nervous 'flight' state ensures the brain keeps flooding the system with stress hormones.

A shallow, rapid breathing pattern and physical tension occur spontaneously when we are under pressure in order to help us make a quick escape and physically protect ourselves if necessary. This is a primitive response to danger not intended to help us take the space with dynamism, charisma and expertise as we perform in a play, sing a song, do a presentation, or go up to the tee in a golf tournament. Centring the breath, however, begins to reverse that stress cycle because the muscle (and therefore emotional) memory of a centred breath is linked to confidence and ease. Breath and mind-set can then work together to create success.

The link between the breath and the mind is fundamental and is encapsulated in the very meaning of the word 'inspiration'. Since ideas arrive with an inspiration of breath, holding the breath can prevent new ideas from forming. When we hold our breath the unconscious mind engages entirely in the effort of trying to make us breathe again. For example when a tough question is fired at someone in a meeting, acute observers will actually see the recipient subtly retract in the area of the diaphragm almost as if he was, indeed, hit by a sharp object in that area. If he then fails to instantly centre the breath, his answer is likely to sound uncertain, the voice may even crack because it is unsupported and the shallow, 'flight' pattern breathing will give him unconfident body language. When he leaves the meeting room and his breath naturally centres, a more effective answer is likely to come flooding into his mind, along with the thought 'Why didn't I say that?!'

Uncentred, held and erratic breathing stops our ability to function under even the slightest pressure. I had an acting student who frustrated his lecturers and directors with his poor listening skills. I observed that he held his breath when an authority figure spoke to him. We worked on releasing his centre and letting his breath drop in, and connected that to listening and letting what was being said to him drop in with his breath. In short, he discovered how to consciously release the muscular holding pattern that stopped his breath. When he began to breathe, he also began to hear!

CONCLUSION

The psycho-physical ramifications of the way in which we breathe affect every aspect of our lives, from physical health to emotional well-being. Shallow breathing affects health in a variety of ways. It pumps less oxygen into the bloodstream and maintains a higher level of stale air in the lungs leading to an increased likelihood of coughs, colds and related infections. It also leads to increased levels of carbon dioxide in the bloodstream, which is one of the physiological causes of anxiety. The way in which we breathe also directly affects levels of confidence and self-esteem, and profoundly influences the more public aspects of our lives as communicators, social beings and 'performers' in our professional lives.

Breathing is intimately connected to the way in which we inhabit our bodies. It affects every aspect of body and vocal language and influences both the way we feel and the way in which others view and react to us. It also determines how well we handle pressure and how easily we bounce back from all that life throws our way. A centred breath will give rise to a supported, resonant, confident sounding voice, making us feel more confident as well. Centring the breath gives us the opportunity to function more effectively in spite of our feelings – to control nerves, anxiety and self-doubt and to replace them with a more positive frame of mind which enables us to function from the most capable side of ourselves. Breath is not just the life force, it is also quintessential in shaping the very way we live our lives.

EXERCISES

The following exercises are a helpful way of experiencing a more centred breath and sound. For a more extensive process I highly recommend Kristin Linklater's brilliant book *Freeing The Natural Voice* (Drama Publishers 2006).

Title: Exercise 1

Aim: Relaxation through breath.

- Find a comfortable, relaxed position lying prone on the floor, hands under the forehead so that you are facing down to the floor and the neck is long. Imagine your lungs are in your buttocks and that a little breath could permeate right down to your tailbone. As the breath drops in, feel the gentle rise of the lower back and the tailbone releasing down towards the floor and as the breath drops out feel the lower back falling and the tailbone rising slightly. If you find this difficult to feel, place a thick book on your tailbone/ pelvis and allow your breath, as it drops in, to gently lift the book a little. Once you have experienced this sensation, remove the book and allow that awareness to help you experience this sensation. Then sit upright in a chair with a hard seat, feet flat on the floor. Let your breath drop in and out naturally. It will be quite small and gentle. Allow the jaw to relax. Part the lips slightly so that, as your breath drops in, you can feel a little cold air coming in through the lips. Imagine your lungs are in your buttocks and that, as the air drops in through the lips, a little breath can also drop down to your lower back and sit bones.

| *Title:* | Exercise 2 |
| *Aim:* | To centre the breath. |

- Lying on your back on the floor in semi-supine: your bare feet flat on the floor, your knees up and bent and your arms comfortably out along the floor, palms of the hands gently facing up rather than down onto the floor.

- Allow the jaw to relax. Part the lips slightly so that, as your breath drops in, you can feel a little cold air coming in through the lips. Imagine a large space in your belly. Now imagine a little air could drop into that space in the belly at the same time as you feel it at your lips. Imagine the lower part of your torso is so free and open it's like an empty shell and as the breath enters through the lips and drops into the belly a little of it could waft around the lower part of your torso.

- Imagine the breath could drop down into your buttocks and that a little bit of breath could delineate the shape of your buttocks from the inside. Now imagine a little breath could waft into your hip sockets, allowing them to breathe; and then imagine that the breath could permeate up through your thighs and into your knees, allowing them to breathe.

- Now allow your feet to gently slide out along the floor so that you are lying flat. Think into the soles of your feet and imagine that they could breathe. Then think into the palms of your hands and imagine that a little breath could enter your body through the palms of your hands. Notice the relaxing sensation of your body breathing gently and easily. Allow your mind to notice your free, centred breathing rhythm without changing it in anyway – allowing it to be as small and gentle as it wants to be. A centred breath may occur deep in the body but it doesn't have to be big. Breath only needs to be as big as the demand that is placed upon it and, right now as you are lying on the floor in a relaxed state, your requirement for breath is quite small.

Title:	Exercise 3
Aim:	To understand breath in the body. (Reike Humming: my version of Kristin Linklater's exercise inspired by Reike healing.)

- Lying in semi-supine, close your eyes and place the palms of your hands flat on your face, one on each side of the nose almost as if you were playing 'peek a boo' with a child. Your fingers will be near the top of your forehead, the heels of your hands just above your jaw line and your elbows will be bent and facing up towards the ceiling.

- Using your mind's eye, picture the spaces under your hands: the tunnels of the sinuses, the large space in the mouth and an enormous, cavernous space at the back of the throat. Allow the jaw muscles to melt and relax and allow the jaw to drop open. As your breath drops in, feel a little cold air coming in through the lips and hitting the gum ridge just behind the top teeth. Imagine the dome of the roof of your mouth is like the high ceiling in a huge cathedral and that the roof of your mouth could almost reach up, cathedral-like, into the top of your skull.

- Picture a huge space between the back of your tongue and the back of your throat and your throat as a very wide, open channel. Imagine it widens further as it reaches down to the very base of your torso.

- Become aware of your breath and the space deep in your body it drops into. Allow a sigh of relief on breath to pour from your belly through the spaces under your hands. Then sigh that relief on sound. Now allow an easy hum on sound to pour up from your belly and out through those spaces in your face and into your hands. Repeat this hum three or four times.

- Then place one hand gently around the front of your throat and the other around the back of your neck. Picture the space between your hands and imagine a very wide, open channel in your throat. Allow a sigh of relief on breath to pour out from the depths of your breathing centre, through that very wide, open channel in your throat and into the spaces in the face and head. Then allow a sigh of relief on sound to pour out on sound. Now allow a hum to pour up from your belly and up through the wide, open channel in your throat and into your face and head. Repeat this hum three or four times.

- Place your hands gently on your upper chest and over your heart. Allow a sigh of relief on breath to pour any feelings in your chest out through your heart and the spaces in the upper chest. Imagine the sigh of relief releases the upper chest, almost allowing it to float up and away with the sigh. Then allow the sigh of relief to pour out on sound. Now allow a hum on sound to pour up from your belly and up through the spaces in your upper chest and into your hands. Repeat this hum three or four times.

- Place your hands gently on your solar plexus and lower ribs. Allow any tension in that area to melt away under your hands. Picture the space in the lower ribcage. Allow a sigh of relief on breath to pour out from your solar plexus, then sigh that relief on sound. Now allow a hum on sound to pour up from your belly, through the spaces in your solar plexus and lower ribs and into your hands. Repeat this hum three or four times.

- Place your hands gently on your lower belly. Imagine the spaces in the your lower belly. Feel the breath in your belly and at your solar plexus. Feel your sacrum on the floor. Allow this lower part of your body to be the centre of your breath, feelings and impulses. Imagine there is a lovely, bright sun in your belly, radiating its warmth throughout your body. Feel its energy strengthen in your belly-pelvis-sacrum area. Allow a sigh of relief on breath to pour out through the space in the lower belly. Then sigh that relief on sound. Now allow a hum to pour out from your belly into your hands. Repeat this hum three or four times.

- Now we will connect all the spaces in the body explored so far. Leaving one hand on the belly, place the other hand on your solar plexus. Imagine a connection between the spaces in the belly and the solar plexus/lower ribs. On breath, sigh that connection between the belly and the solar plexus. Then sigh that connection on sound. Then hum that connection, repeating the hum two or three times.

- Leaving one hand on the belly, place the other hand on the front of the throat. Imagine a connection between the belly, the solar plexus, the upper chest and the wide, open channel in the throat. Sigh that connection on breath, then on sound. Then hum that connection, repeating the hum two or three times.

- With one hand on the belly, place the other hand on one side of the face. Imagine a connection between the belly, the solar plexus, the upper chest, the open channel in the throat and the spaces in the face. On breath, sigh that connection from the belly, through all the spaces right up to the face. Then sigh that connection on sound. Then hum that connection, repeating the hum two or three times.

- With one hand on the belly, place the other hand on top of your head. Imagine a connection from the belly, through all the spaces and right up to the top of your head. On breath, sigh this connection. Then sigh that connection on sound. Then hum that connection, repeating the hum two or three times.

- Gently open your eyes, stretch and yawn and sit up. Register what the sensation of the breath and vibrations travelling through the different parts of your body felt like. Were some more intense than others? Were you able to imagine or experience a connection between these areas of your body through your breath and sound?

BIBLIOGRAPHY

Damasio, Antonio (2000) *The Feeling of What Happens.* London: Vintage.

Gershon, Michael (1999) *The Second Brain.* London: HarperPerennial.

Goleman, Daniel (1996) *Emotional Intelligence.* London: Bloomsbury.

Greenfield, Susan (2002) *The Private Life of The Brain.* London: Penguin Books.

Linklater, Kristin (2006) *Freeing The Natural Voice.* Hollywood: Drama Publishers.

O'Connor, J. and Seymour, J. (1994) *Training With NLP.* London: Thorsons.

CHAPTER 7

The Alchemy of Breathing

KRISTIN LINKLATER

There is no one correct way to breathe. There is breathing that works for yoga, breathing that works for swimming, there is the proper breathing for martial arts and the best for playing the trumpet, there is meditation breathing and at least a dozen different 'correct' ways of breathing for singing. Our breathing muscles are multifarious and adaptable. They can perform both voluntarily and involuntarily. Their primary purpose is, of course, to keep us alive; this they do on the involuntary level. My particular interest in breath is the way in which it creates voice as it passes through the vocal folds and how it helps us either to reveal or hide the truth as we speak. The role played by breathing in the art of acting has occupied me professionally for 50 years and, in the art of acting, the goals are believability and a sense of limitlessness. We search for truth in the language of extremity and in the most intimate emotional expression. The alchemy of inspired communication is a mix of emotion, intellect and voice. The 'prima materia' is breath. This fundamental element of truthful speaking is accessible for anyone involved in speaking publicly – or indeed privately.

How do you experience the alchemy and art of breathing for voice? My starting point is to pay attention to the centre of the diaphragm and, with the lips slightly apart, to tune in to the rhythm of natural, everyday breathing allowing the outgoing breath to escape over the lips in a small loose puff of air 'ff'.

Then, in my teaching, I break down the sophisticated geography of the breathing mechanism to:

Diaphragm and solar plexus for sensitivity and emotional connection
Pelvic floor and sacrum for instinct and power
Intercostals for capacity.

Of course all these should act together in sublime collaboration on the involuntary level. Voluntarily the best contribution we can make is to create fertile conditions for the intricately coordinated activity that delivers accurate communication (thought into word; brain-waves into sound-waves: through breath). We need to get out of the way. But in order to get out of the way we must be able to see the way – we must get to know our breathing process.

The first step toward this knowledge is to be able to train the mind's eye accurately on the diaphragm, intercostals and pelvic floor. However, mere anatomical accuracy isn't enough to effect the alchemical transformation that makes breath serve the goal of truthful speaking. The senses, imagination and imagery must be accessories in our breath quest if brain and body are to unite in expressiveness. No neat anatomical diagram of your breathing apparatus will help – indeed such a diagram is impossible, there's nothing neat about either breathing or the art of speaking. Here's a word picture instead:

The tapestry of the breathing musculature wraps around the inside of the ribcage, billows into the diaphragm (that great elastic dome that forms a floor to the lungs and a ceiling to the stomach) laces down by the lumbar spine and weaves its way through the webbing of the pelvic floor among the muscles and nerves of its genital neighbours. These interior muscles coordinate in opening the air sacs in the lungs (as the diaphragm drops down) so that breath rushes in, and closing them (as the diaphragm moves up) so that breath releases out. This is breathing for living.

When the impulse to speak sparks the circuitry of nerves that cohabit with the breathing muscles, the interaction between breath and vocal folds creates vibrations of sound. Then sound is moulded into words by the lips and the tongue.

Breath is the key to restoring the deepest connections with impulse, with emotion, with imagination and thereby with language. The voice is not just a musical instrument to be played skilfully – it is a human instrument.

Reconditioning the way the voice works means reconditioning breathing processes on deep levels of involuntary neuro-physiological, psycho-physical, brain-body functioning. Any serious practice of breath and voice must bring to the level of consciousness activities that normally belong in the unconscious sector of daily being.

Hard as that may seem, guidance is very much at hand. Look long at a small baby's breathing and observe how biological impulses govern the movements of breath. A baby's breathing is arrhythmic. When a hungry baby approaches the breast you may see a thrill ripple through the almost transparent body while the anticipation of assuagement excites the breath into panting. These first biological experiences imprint the infant organism. As the baby matures the organism absorbs increasingly complex sensory impressions and eventually registers emotions varying through the graduated degrees of all the passions.

And then nurture takes nature in hand. Spontaneous emotional expression must be suppressed for a well-ordered society to be maintained. In the family from the age of about three and later in school we unconsciously impose controls that subvert the involuntary breathing process. The baby's primary neuro-physiological experience is: 'I breathe, I live; I wail, I survive.' Then it transforms to: 'If I wail, I'll die; if I hold my breath and suppress what I feel, I'll survive.'

We can learn from babies and we can learn from actors – good ones! Audiences love actors who are believable, untrammelled by convention, emotionally and imaginatively daring and – let's say, transparent: as transparent as babies but with the knowledge and life experience of adults.

If we are born with feelings and the voice to convey them, then the question arises as to when, how and why we have modified the direct expression of emotion. When, how and why did our mode of speaking evolve? Do we remember being told to 'be quiet – speak nicely' when we were four or five years old? Do we recall being told not to giggle or shout in the classroom? Do any men remember 'big boys don't cry' as an admonition? Do you remember being sent out of the room when you erupted in rage at your parents? Many of us developed a mode of speaking in our teens when we wanted to speak in the same way as the 'in' crowd. Does the way you speak reflect your family, your region, your profession, your favourite celebrity? We learned how to modify our vocal expression. And the final questions may be: 'Is this really my voice? Can I find my real voice?'

Recovery of voice begins with recovery of breathing. If I am interested in rediscovering the authenticity of my voice and thereby a deeper authentic self, I must start with an awareness of my breathing habits. Most people know that the diaphragm is the primary breathing muscle and that it forms a domed floor for the lungs and ceiling for the stomach, cutting the torso in two horizontally. We may also know that the diaphragm cannot be moved voluntarily and yet we must activate change in the behaviour of this involuntary breathing muscle. For any speaker who wishes to explore the rich inner realm of breathing, imagery is the key to the adventure and the art. Our autonomic organism is governed by sensory imagery. Unconsciously our breathing patterns have been conditioned by sensory imagery – new, conscious imagery can dissolve those patterned habits.

This is how I introduce the awareness of natural breathing:

First comes physical awareness, with particular attention paid to the spine as the two-way message channel between brain and body and the essential support for the three main areas of breathing musculature – diaphragm, inner abdominals (or crura/psoas – those lacey connections from diaphragm to pelvic floor) and intercostals. Then we observe the diaphragm, and pay attention to the natural breathing rhythm – without organizing it. The mouth is a little bit open so that the outgoing breath arrives in the front of the mouth forming a small 'ff'. Picture the centre of the diaphragm – it drops as the breath enters – then the breath immediately escapes out – then there is a tiny pause, a moment of nothing (not a holding) – then you feel breath wanting to enter again and all you do is *yield* to that need. You don't have to breathe in – breath will enter. Let it happen – let the air breathe you. When we're relaxed our bodies only need a very small exchange of air in order to stay alive.

The words 'inhale' and 'exhale' are banished. They are active verbs and the diaphragm is a passive (reactive) muscle. The language of breath awareness replaces control verbs with release messages. 'Allow the breath to enter', 'let the breath drop in', 'feed in a sigh impulse and then let it release out', 'open inside for the breath to come in – then let it escape'. This vocabulary gradually builds mental freedom, dissolving protective habits in the mind and the body. We are getting out of the way and beginning to see the way.

One must not assume that internal imaging is easy. Many people feel faint when first asked to close their eyes and picture their skeletons. And the instruction: 'Picture the movement of your diaphragm as you breathe; now model that movement with your hands' gives rise to an astonishing display of mimed balloons, bellows, jellyfish and concertinas. Beginners cannot at first see the down and up movement that draws breath in on descent and releases it on ascent. Gradually the inner eye learns to see, as it were, in the dark and gradually the inner landscape is illuminated so that diaphragm, spine, ribs, pelvis, sacrum, tailbone and organs become familiar, visible territory. As long as the physical breathing experience is dominated by the obvious out and in, forward and back movement of the abdominal wall the true movement of the diaphragm remains invisible. Two messages must be given:

Relax the abdominal wall

Picture the vertical movement of the diaphragm.

The first instruction is executed consciously, the second is conveyed through the body-mind's eye.

Consciously giving up habitual breath control can be a frightening mind-body moment. Habits of holding and controlling the breath are often set in moments of terror, in moments when the body knew it was dangerous to feel and express emotion. Sadly, many of these habits are set in childhood under traumatic circumstances.

Louisa, who is in her 40s, said:

> You invited me to relax my breathing and my jaw... and the fact of allowing the breath just to 'be' revived emotions that had been suffocated, that all these muscles have learned to repress. I heard something like a new voice. It wasn't my habitual voice, it was more alive, the sound more extroverted, easy, much more in contact with my desire to communicate. My heart felt opened. Paying attention to my breath was a medicine for fear.

Sometimes when someone relaxes and the breath drops deeper in the body tears will flow. There may be no apparent reason for the tears, no story to tell, it's just a relief for the body to let go of its habitual protection and allow emotion and breath to reconnect as they are designed to do.

Observe your breathing habits during an ordinary day. When do you hold your breath? Why? Fear? Anxiety? Boredom? Insecurity? The body-mind may unconsciously be trying not to 'fall apart' saying 'you've got to keep yourself together' – quite unnecessarily! What happens when you relax and let yourself breathe in difficult circumstances? Almost always, contrary to the body's expectation, relaxed breathing results not in tears, not in falling apart, but in a feeling of confidence and intelligence. And you can support your breathing awareness with imaginative input. Picture your solar plexus in the centre of your diaphragm, your own solar system, an inner sun, bringing warmth and light, unifying the experience of emotion and breath and thought, as though your brain were in your belly.

From the small 'ff' of the natural breathing rhythm a sigh will inevitably be born. We need to sigh. When we sigh we satisfy an organic impulse that needs *more*. The body signals its need for more oxygen. And now our breathing exercises embrace sighing. A sigh is a bigger impulse. A sigh is often pleasurable. Even when a sigh is filled with sorrow it is also filled with relief that the sorrow can be expressed and that is a kind of pleasure. Introducing the sigh to different parts of the body begins the exploration of instinct, power and capacity.

When we continue the exploration of breathing while lying on the floor we start to stimulate the diaphragmatic crura connections through the psoas muscles by way of the lumbar vertebrae to the pelvic floor. These crura are muscles deep inside the torso that form part of the psoas system which is a great triangular core of support muscles for the lower spine, pelvis and hips. If we think of feeding a sigh impulse way down into the hip sockets and the pelvic basin, breath does not actually go there. But the impulse galvanizes the crura muscles that run from the diaphragm along the lumbar spine and the sacrum to the pelvic musculature. The beautiful triangular sacrum bone is threaded with nerves that weave their way throughout the pelvic region sparking the sacral and sexual nerve centres. This is the home of instinct, intuition and, dare I suggest, the creative impulse.

A sigh impulse that travels through these nether regions engages the crura muscles which help to draw the diaphragm deeply down bringing huge volumes of breath to the lungs and releasing energies throughout the body that have lain dormant. Imagery will trigger this breathing experience rather than sheer anatomical persuasion.

Haerry, a talented Korean actress, described her discovery of the deeper realm of her breathing thus:

> I remember the first time I felt the rush of air coming into my body. Up to that point, my idea of picturing my body was very literal. I always saw my body as dense, filled with organs, muscles and so on. After we spent about an hour on the floor, you led us through the image of an open throat going all the way down through the body. With that picture, I suddenly emptied out my thought and my literal picture of the inside of my body. A weight in my chest lifted. Right then, like a fresh waterfall, a rush of air dropped in and it was something I had never felt before. I know if I had tried to rationalize how I was going to take in a bigger breath, it would never have happened. Once my body was introduced to that experience, I knew my breath was not something that was controlled by my intellect only.

These connections are primal. They plug us into our instincts and our power.

An unvoiced sigh is all feeling: relief. A voiced sigh starts to engage thought. A sigh with words is equal parts feeling and thought. It can be said that voice picks up emotion and speech picks up thoughts. Emotion must be freely expressible if thoughts are to be freely expressed. But habits of repression and inhibition often block the initial desire to communicate. A sigh of relief undoes both physical and mental restrictions.

We can sigh a story out and communicate not only information but the emotional colours of the story – sometimes these colours are in rich oils, sometimes in pastels, sometimes there's a wash of colour/emotion, sometimes it's just in black and white. The words in one's head are full of the inflections of colour.

In my first description of the breathing apparatus I invoked the image of a tapestry woven around the inner walls of the body. It can help to know that the root of the word 'text' (as in the text of a story) is the same as the root of the word 'tapestry': both words originate in the Latin 'tessere' which means 'to weave'. Now, therefore, you can let the words (the stitches?) of your story be sewn into the fibre of your breathing and your voice will be filled with living pictures.

At first, a sigh may result in a somewhat collapsing physique – the ribs sink and there is a downward feeling. But once the experience has become familiar we can pay attention to the fact that despite the collapse of the ribs the diaphragm 'whooshes' upward through the ribcage on the out-sigh.

Then we practise sighing standing up with hands on head, ribs floating wide, with a clear picture of the sigh/whoosh fountaining up and out. This immediately results in a feeling of dynamism and energy. The unvoiced, voiced and verbalized sigh/whoosh let go upward and outward. The 'letting-go' is akin to archery: the ingoing thought-feeling-breath impulse is the bowstring drawing back, the brain lets go of the impulse (the fingers let go of the bowstring) and the words (the arrow) fly to the listener (the target).

Sighing is a device for letting go and not controlling the manner of communication. Once you let go of physical control your job is to think and feel clearly. This works as well for singing as for speaking.

Here again is Louisa:

it was a long exercise with arpeggios, lying on the floor, changing positions, going up and down on pitches... and I absolutely didn't like my voice. I felt it stuck, there was so much tension. I felt miserable because I was failing. But I decided to focus all my attention on breathing, trying not to make a more beautiful sound but to sigh it from me, from my inside without caring about the resultant sound. I let the sound of the piano drop down into my belly and sighed it out easily. And I slowly started enjoying the exercise. As long as I was focused on sighing my voice found different paths, new resonances. Being focused on breath instead of on the final result of sound was extraordinarily helpful, specially when we reached higher pitches. Usually I can't reach them and they were just there.

For singers I strongly recommend singing while lying face down on the floor – hands under the forehead, sighing from the lower back. Sighing arpeggios in many adapted yoga positions, on all-fours, hanging upside down, with arm-swings, gradually makes the whole respiratory event elastic. Small sighs, medium sighs, big sighs condition the breathing apparatus to experience short thoughts sparking short breaths, medium-length thoughts for medium breaths and big, long thoughts inspiring deep big breaths.

Once respiratory action has been fully exercised with big sighs of pleasurable relief it can respond to huge impulses of rage, grief and terror and still operate on the principle of release. For actors this is an essential extension of the philosophy of the sigh. What a relief for Lear to bellow at the storm! What a relief for Oedipus to roar his pain! What a relief for Constance to mourn her son!

While the next breathing exploration is, perhaps, of particular interest for the actor, there may well be adventurous souls who would like the stretch in vocal and respiratory demand as we now pay more attention to the ribs, the whole chest, the intercostals. Capacity. When the emotion is big and the thought is long there is a greater demand on lung capacity. The diaphragm drops deeper, the ribcage opens more palpably and because the lungs go down further in the back than in the front, the opening of the back ribs is the most important part of ribcage response. Capacity is natural and built-in to the anatomy. We have to stimulate it imaginatively.

The movement of the back-ribs and side-ribs can be most vividly appreciated when one is lying on one's belly on the floor, head turned to one side, arms down by the sides. Sighing. On the in-breath the lumbar spine can be felt to lengthen while the tailbone moves toward the floor and the lower back-ribs widen. The injunction: 'Back-belly-side-ribs' on each big new ingoing breath-thought restores respiratory vigor. So long as the instigating thought is clear the outgoing breath can still be trusted to perform its task with the encouragement of: 'Let go, sigh it out; don't hold on; open up for the breath to come in; let the thought drop deep inside; release the thought.' The thought might be one arpeggio, then two, then three. Then six big lines of Shakespeare.

'Back-belly-side-ribs' awareness can be practised on all-fours, squatting, hanging head downward, slowly coming to an upright position. It is the content of the thought that controls the breath and makes it last as long as necessary. With a developing mentality of freedom the involuntary breath processes re-establish themselves in unity with sensory feeling and emotional impulse. All you have to say to yourself is 'Open'. This becomes the new natural breathing experience. You have a choice in what you want to express, you are no longer under the limiting dictatorship of habit and, according to your impulse and your choice, your breath will tell your truth. You are the alchemist in charge of the prima materia that transmutes thought into words.

Counter-productive terms for alchemical breathing include: breath *control*, breath *support*, breath *management*. Advancing science has shown (with the use, for instance, of ultrasound imaging) many muscle levels that engage in the respiratory event. They are engaged naturally from the intrinsic involuntary activity if the integrity of the psycho-physical approach is maintained. Using such anatomical knowledge to control breathing and voice is counter-productive because it interferes with the sensory-emotional connection.

Susan, while training to be a voice teacher, made this observation of a class she had taught on breath capacity:

> I wanted my students to think of themselves as 'pulmonary athletes', a phrase I had borrowed from someone who teaches vocal anatomy for singers. You invited me to think about 'pulmonary artist' as an adjustment. I think that phrase conjures a much better picture of the work of the involuntary breathing musculature. The word 'artist' by one definition is 'somebody who does something with great skill and creativity'. Certainly using our imagination in order to stimulate the intercostals is a creative skill. From golf umbrellas and trampolines to trolls living under the bridges of the rib bones, imagistic thought really works. Maybe to be a pulmonary artist is to be stimulated into creative thought, which in turn activates our involuntary breathing system.

I must end with a caveat – images are powerful, imagination even more so. Images and imagination have equal creative and destructive power. There are creative images, there are inspiring images and there are shocking, counter-productive images; there are utilitarian images which deaden the impulse connection (pistons, and, prevalent in the voice science field, the image of a turkey baster – aesthetically offensive on many levels) and there are images that enliven the sense of self that should come with all breath work – let's call that 'breath play'.

Images, imagination, organic breathing are exercised to serve everyday speaking and public performance. Shakespeare gives us the incentive and the necessity:

> Speak what we feel, not what we ought to say.
>
> Edgar: King Lear Act V sc 3

I will speak as liberal as the north.

Let heaven and man and devils, let them all,

All, all cry shame upon me, yet I'll speak.

Emilia: Othello Act V sc 2

And, in response to an injunction to hold her peace, Constance says:

No, no, I will not, having breath to cry.

O that my tongue were in the thunder's mouth,

Then with a passion would I shake the world.

King John Act III sc 4

EXERCISE

Title:	Kindling the breath
Aim:	This is an advanced exercise to develop responsiveness, strength, agility and flexibility in the whole breathing apparatus. (Not for beginners. It will only work for those who have spent time exploring the basic relaxation exercises that lead to a clear picture of the involuntary breathing process.)
	Of prime importance in this exercise is to know the difference between a sigh and a big breath. A big breath is empty air; a sigh contains feeling generated by a thought-feeling impulse.
How often:	You can do this any time you feel the need for breath and brain energy.

• Prepare by stretching, yawning, relaxing down and up the spine, shaking loose.

All the following exercises are to be practised with the mouth slightly open and the breath arriving in the front of the mouth.

• Picture your whole torso from front to back, from side to side, pelvis to shoulders as though it were a great elastic container. Into the centre of the container feed four huge impulses for four huge sighs of pleasurable relief one after the other without pausing in between. Let the impulse move the breath and the breath move the body from inside out. The breath fills you from the bottom up. Picture the ingoing sigh-breath as if it were water filling a jug from the bottom up and the outgoing sigh-breath falling out suddenly as though the jug were tipped upside down and all the water falls out at once.

• Rest.

Create and re-create the impulse – do not just repeat the big breath.

- Repeat the process, re-creating the four huge sigh impulses and this time picture what is happening to the diaphragm. Imagine it as a silky, billowing parachute shape being blown downward by the ingoing sigh-breath and blown upward from below by the outgoing sigh-breath.

- Rest.

- Now explore feeding in six smaller faster impulses of relief that affect a more central part of the diaphragm-parachute – about the size of a frisbee. These are medium-sized sighs of relief. Your job is to create and re-create the six relief impulses. Let the seventh impulse trigger a big sigh, allow all the breath to escape and then gently be restored.

- Exercise your ability to re-create repeated impulses of relief without their becoming shallow, thoughtless or mechanical.

You may find yourself getting a bit dizzy as you do this. Always rest between the clusters of sigh-breath impulses. Eventually you will be able to do these exercises without dizziness. Your breathing stamina will have developed and your system will be able to cope with the increased oxygen intake.

- Now focus your attention on the very centre of the dome of the diaphragm. Feed in many, many quick, lively impulses of pleasurable anticipation that flutter tiny breaths in and out of that centre. The anticipation stimulates the breath and the breath flutters the centre of the diaphragm. Tiny breaths fly in and out, fast and loose. Then there is a transitional impulse that results in a final sigh of relief.

- Leave the outside abdominal muscles really loose; make sure they are not making the movements. They will be moved from inside but should not get tight at any point. The breath goes in and out evenly; that is, you should not get fuller as you go on, nor should your lungs get emptier in the course of the exercise.

- Agility and flexibility increase and the breathing muscles learn to remain free of tension while intensity builds. The picture of a puppy, happy to go for a walk, is a good model for the quick, light anticipation panting of the final part of the exercise. There is no tension in the outer belly of that puppy.

All the above exercises can be practised hanging head downward, lying on one's back or belly on the floor, on all-fours and, once the relaxation and flexibility are established, standing, with hands clasped on top of the head. This position (making sure the spine remains long) helps to lift the ribs and encourages the diaphragm to 'whoosh' up through the ribcage and breath to release dynamically upward and outward.

See *Freeing the Natural Voice: Imagery and Art in the Practice of Voice and Language* by Kristin Linklater for preparatory exercises and more detail.

BIBLIOGRAPHY

Linklater, Kristin (2006) *Freeing the Natural Voice: Imagery and Art in the Practice of Voice and Language.* London: Nick Hern Books.

SECTION 3

Breath and Holistic Practice

JANE BOSTON AND RENA COOK

An extended gaze eastwards has been incorporated into western performance praxis for the greater part of the twentieth century onwards, in part to refresh and revalue its own moribund traditions. The origin of this gaze is complex but its recent incarnation relates in part to the liberation philosophies of the 1960s with their reaction to the authoritarian structures and materialistic values of the previous decade. This gave rise to a myriad of 'new' thinking about established orthodoxies that were mirrored by many involved with the theory and practices of performance. These all shared similar cultural origins, reflected a West to East gaze and were almost exclusively holistic in nature.

Tara McAllister-Viel takes us eastwards with her subtle account of the ways in which the dualistic thinking embedded in western philosophy may have limited the conceptualization of the breath. She examines the place of breath in relation to the body–mind dichotomies and invites us to adopt a different and more holistic approach informed by other cultural practices and values. Interweaving her own cultural background in the States with those discovered in Korea, she offers specific observations about the ways in which the arts of Dahnjeon breathing can provide efficient muscular use as a foundation for good breath and vocal use.

As well as looking to the Far East, the gaze has also gone specifically to the indigenous cultures of the world. The chapter by Marj McDaid draws upon Central and Eastern Europe where she explores the evolution of her own breathing practice based on the influence of the Eastern Siberian teacher Nelly Dougar-Zhabon whose practice involves not only the influence of Siberian shamanism, but also Tibetan Dynamic Meditation and Qi Gong. An approach based upon a synthesis of methods, with reference to their specific implications for actor training processes, forms the basis of this chapter.

Michael Morgan follows with an exploration of the ways in which the exterior forms of of Chinese Qi Gong, such as acupuncture, martial arts, stretching and massage and the interior forms, such as a range of internal breathing methods, can relate to western mindbody training. He suggests that 'questions, rather than answers' should provide the most fruitful starting point for this complex examination involving forms that have been cultivated in one context and then transplanted to another.

Debbie Green, in an account of the evolution of her movement practice, places importance on the sensual activity of the breath. She instructively concludes that this, too, will vary between practices: 'the movement we do on the out-breath in Pilates or Bartenieff Fundamentals may well be different from those we do in Yoga, but in any of these, connection to personal breath is key'. Whilst her focus begins with the actor, it is clearly relevant to all who work with the body from an intercultural and an interdisciplinary perspective. Her focus on the core energy of the breath suggests that everyone can access and benefit from it, creating a sense of multi-dimensionality where 'the outside (is) informed by the inside through the breath' (Green).

Rena Cook looks specifically at the healing methodologies of the East in order to reinvigorate the breathing practices of the western academies that have become stale and reliant on old mechanistic models and interrogates the question of 'authenticity' within both presence and performance. Where the more traditional western practices have been seen by some to be tainted with outmoded thought and knowledge, an account is provided as to why it has been to the older, deemed more 'spiritual', practices of the East that many practitioners have turned. Here, where they have found a more convincing unity of heart and mind, it is seen that the breath can provide a crucial meeting point between the conscious and the unconscious mind and offer synthesis rather than division.

CHAPTER 8

Dahnjeon Breathing

TARA McALLISTER-VIEL

Breathing through 'dahnjeon(s)' is a way of breathing that can be found in many different Asian modes of training. The particular exercise called 'Dahnjeon Breathing' found at the end of this chapter is an exercise adapted from my experiences of long-term, rigorous study of several Asian practices.[1] Regular practice with these exercises will help you create efficient muscular use as the foundation for good breath and voice production. Long-term, rigorous practice will help you cultivate ki (energy), which will give your sound a sense of strength beyond muscular strength. These exercises will also provide the foundation for creating a sense of being in the here and now and help create the necessary preparation for drawing in your listener and

---

1   My experiences include training in hatha yoga, taijichuan (Wu form) and a South Indian martial art called kalarippayattu under Phillip Zarrilli as part of my MFA-Acting (three year) degree, Asian/ Experimental Theatre Program, University of Wisconsin-Madison, USA. For a better understanding of the way I learned taijichuan (Wu form) as adapted for acting training, see the writings of A.C. Scott, specifically *Actors are madmen*, Madison: University of Wisconsin Press, 1982. For an understanding of the way I trained in kalarippayattu as part of my acting training, see the writings of Phillip Zarrilli, specifically *When the body becomes all eyes: paradigms, discourses and practices of power in Kalarippayattu, a South Indian martial art*, Oxford: Oxford University Press, 1998; and *From Kalarippayattu to Beckett* (Video recording), Exeter: Arts Documentation Unit, 1999. I returned to study again under Zarrilli during my (four-year) PhD-Performance Practice (Voice) degree, University of Exeter, England. I have also had private study in a traditional Korean vocal art form called p'ansori over the course of four years in Seoul, Korea, with Human Cultural Treasures Han Nong Son and Song UHyang, and additional study with p'ansori practitioner/actress Choi Yoon Chul at The Korean National University of Arts, School of Drama, and p'ansori practitioner/scholar Dr Chan E. Park, at her home in Columbus, Ohio. I have also studied seated meditation at Wa Gye Sa temple (Korea).

sustaining communication. Before you begin the exercise sequence, it is important to understand:

- What is dahnjeon(s)?

- How breathing from the (lower) dahnjeon helps train the voice?

- How using this breathing practice can benefit your voice training?

WHAT IS A 'DAHNJEON'?

Sometimes 'dahnjeon' is translated into English as 'centre', or 'energy centre' (Benedetti 1990, p.28–9). Dahnjeon(s) are a part of an eastern understanding of the body integral to eastern medicinal praxis and fundamental to the way the body functions. There are three internal dahnjeons and four external dahnjeons. The 'lower dahnjeon' also referred to as dantien or tan-den (Japan) or nabhi mula (Sanskrit meaning 'the root of the navel'),[2] is located two inches below the navel and two inches inside the body. The 'middle dahnjeon' is located two inches inside the body behind the sternum, and the 'upper dahnjeon', is located roughly between and just above the eyes within the forehead (also referred to in some Asian practices as the 'mind's eye', the 'inner eye' or 'third eye'). There are four external dahnjeons, one located in the palm of each hand where the centre fingernail touches the palm while fisting (*jangshim* in Korean) and one located on the bottom of each foot, just below the ball when the foot is flexed (*yongchun* in Korean).[3]

This body knowledge becomes the foundation for the transmission of embodied practices. Because the exercise at the end of this chapter focuses on the lower dahnjeon, I will concentrate on this area in order to better explain one understanding of how a dahnjeon can function in developing the breath for sounding.

THE LOWER DAHNJEON AND TRAINING THE VOICE

Sometimes the lower dahnjeon as an 'energy centre' is compared to a western understanding of 'centre of gravity' in the body because both are formless and invisible but have palpable physiological effects on the body (Benedetti 1990, p.28–9). However,

---

2   Difference in the spelling of dahnjeon into English has been influenced by the Korean government's adoption of a new spelling system July, 2000. The Ministry of Culture and Tourism (MOCT) introduced the MOCT Hangeul Romanization System to replace the formerly used McCune-Reischauer system. Also, different spellings in English are adapted from other languages using various other spelling approaches.

3   My understandings of 'dahnjeon' are based in Korean practices. Yuasa Yasuo provides other understandings of 'dantian' [Chinese] or 'tanden' [Japanese] meditative and self-cultivation practices refer to Yuasa 1993, p.79.

the lower dahnjeon works differently from centre of gravity. Breathing through the lower dahnjeon trains the mind through the body, cultivating an intense bodymind relationship and 'ki' (Korea), also referred to as 'chi' (China) 'qi' (Japan), 'prana' or 'pranavayu' (India). Ki moves in/through/around the bodymind through 'dahnjeons' and a system of channels called 'meridians' (*kyung lack* in Korean), travelling down the back of the body (*yang* energy) and up the front of the body (*eum* or *yin* energy) in a cyclical process, alternating between eum-yang polarities in the body (Yuasa 1993, p.75–6; Yoo in *CTR* 2007, p.87).

When breathing through the lower dahnjeon while voicing, the resultant sound manifests a sense of strength that cannot be explained through the body's muscularity alone.[4] Abdominal muscle(s) are used in combination with breathing energy or ki, creating a strong resonant sound that is compelling to listen to.

DAHNJEON BREATHING AND TRAINING THE VOICE THROUGH BODYMIND

Sometimes the energy of the breath can be understood through training metaphors. Here, I am referring to breathing energy, or ki, as a physical reality and material condition of training and performance. Not only can the practitioner feel this energy, sometimes recognized as heat or vibrations, but the listener can hear within the sound a concentration of focused awareness during communication.

One use of breath/ki for the practitioner is to prepare and sustain the breath for sounding. To better understand how this might work, we can find insights from one of the earliest explanations. Zeami Motokiyo (1364–1443), in his treatise *Kakyo*, discussed how ki functioned when training the Japanese Noh actor's voice, 'First the Key; Second the Activating Force (chi); Third, the Voice.' Mark Nearman explains his interpretation of Zeami's instruction,

> That which inwardly must receive, preserve and sustain tonal pitch is identified as the actor's *ch'i*. Before attempting to vocalize, an actor should first listen to the sound of the flute or in the case of a student, the teacher's voice.

4   P'ansori scholar Um Hae-Kyung wrote in her description of how the (lower) dahnjeon functions, 'pressure is exerted on the diaphragm in combination with dantian respiration to push out the vocal sound more powerfully. The dantian respiration makes the most of breathing energy supported and controlled by the abdominal muscle around the umbilicus and lower abdomen' (Um 1992, p.128). Dr Um is specifically referring to the function of the dahnjeon in the principle p'ansori vocal technique of t'ongsong (lit. straight voice) or chungangsong (lit. central or principle voice). Similarly, 'breathing energy' is described by p'ansori practitioner and scholar Dr Chan E. Park as resonating 'with ki (strength)' which 'is said to resonate in the lower abdomen (Park 2003, p.157).'

On the basis of that externally produced tonality, the actor should determine his 'tonal center,' by 'hearing' and sustaining it within his own mind. He experiences that tone as 'vibrating' within himself, particularly in his tanden (dahnjeon). The performer then 'closes his eyes,' that is, he concentrates on that tonal center to the exclusion of all external 'visual' stimuli, and inhales. Only when he has gone through this process is he ready to 'open his mouth and begin to vocalize.' (Nearman in *Monumenta Nipponica*, 1982, p.347)

Listening to a sound and sustaining it before reproducing it might be understood in western practice as 'ear-training'. But in Zeami's description the practitioner sustains the tone in his 'mind'. Something other than the ear is being trained. The mind is being trained through the body. Sometimes the lower dahnjeon is understood as the 'seat of the mind.' This is very different from a western way of understanding 'mind' and its relationship to the body and how breath can actualize this relationship.

The most fundamental difference between eastern and western views of 'mind' begin with the relationship between the body and the mind. American philosopher Thomas P. Kasulis suggests that although classical Greek philosophers examined the distinction between mind and body, René Descartes is responsible for an ontological difference between mind and body. He argues that this division was an essential step in separating the values of religious thought from science and mathematics and helped establish the modern western worldview (Kasulis 1993, p.xvi–xviii).

Historically in the East, the human body is understood as a medium of practical experience, realized through a unity of body and mind. This bodymind unity is as fundamental to an eastern worldview as mind–body dualism is fundamental to the West. As a philosophy and practice, perhaps 'bodymind' can be mapped throughout Asia, most probably beginning in India and travelling to China, Korea and Japan through the practice of Buddhism. Unlike western monastic tradition, the bodymind in eastern ideology must be integrated in order to understand the 'self' or 'true self'. In Japanese Buddhist self-cultivation methods, monks traditionally trained the body as a means to enlightenment. The body was not neglected but cultivated as a means to achieving spirituality.

The fundamental difference between western and eastern philosophies of the body gave rise to methodological differences in training the body/voice. Japanese philosopher Yuasa Yasuo wrote,

In short, the mind that is subject dominates and moves the body that is object and this is conscious bodily movement. In the state of body–mind oneness, the mind moves while unconsciously becoming one with the body. That is, there is no longer a felt distinction between the mind qua subject and the body qua object; the subject is simultaneously the object and the object is simultaneously the subject. The movement of the object that is the body is such that it is wholly the movement of the mind that is subject . . .Zeami calls this state 'no-mind' (*mushin*) or 'emptiness' (*ku*). (1993, p.28)

The mind and the body become one through the practice of training the body, through the process of embodying a practice. The practice itself, whether in my various experiences training in a traditional Korean vocal art called p'ansori, cultivating seated meditation at Wa gye sa (temple) in Seoul, or 'moving' mediation in martial arts, the set of skills being developed are dependent upon bodymind oneness. It is the fundamental means by which other skills in each of these various practices can be accomplished.

THE BENEFIT OF CULTIVATING 'NO-MIND' INTO 'VOCAL PRESENCE'

From my different trainings, I understand 'no-mind' to be the experience of performing a task in the present moment, when my mind and body are in the same space and time together. 'No-mind' is not 'zoning out' or behaving in an 'unconscious' manner, but is a kind of focus, attention or 'heightened awareness'.

As an example, during a daily activity like tying my shoe I perform this task habitually, most probably through muscle memory recall. Perhaps this habit is 'unconscious' because I do not have to 'think' about it. But when I transfer that same activity in front of an audience of on-lookers, the daily task of tying my shoe becomes what Eugenio Barba might call 'extra-daily' (Barba and Savarese 1991). I am no longer just tying my shoe but performing the act of tying my shoe in front of others. The performance of tying my shoe involves more concentration and focus. If tying my shoe in my private life was 'unconscious response', when I am in front of an audience I have a heightened awareness of this task and am conscious of it as a performer. If the task appears 'unconscious' or 'natural' it is because I have trained my body to fulfil this aesthetic expectation. But I am not 'unconscious' or unaware of this activity during its performance on-stage. I am using bodymind unity to focus my concentration on the task so that it is performed with 'no-mind', my mind and body are together in this space and together in this performative moment, without the self-consciousness of pointing to the task as a performance.

Achieving 'no-mind' through breathing from the dahnjeon can also prepare and sustain a connection with the audience. For philosopher and physician Drew Leder, 'forming one body', a major principle in the Neo-Confucian worldview, is a process that creates a 'profound interconnection between body and world (and) invites an ontology and ethics of interconnection' (1990, p.161). Leder wrote in regards to Zen meditation,

> The meditator finds that he or she 'is breathed' as much as the breather. Watching the breath come in and go out for minutes or hours, one is saturated by the presence of a natural power that outruns the 'I.' Breathing simply happens and happens and happens. There is no need for willful management; all is accomplished without effort on one's part. Thus breathing becomes the very prototype of Zen/Taoist *wu-wei*, literally translated as 'non-action.' This term refers to the effortless acting typical of one who has broken free from ego-identification. (1990, p.171)

In Asian practice, the training of the breath may begin with the physical awareness of the body breathing but after long-term practice the practitioner experiences an 'energy flow' independent of the physical process of breathing (Nearman in *Monumenta Nimpponica* 1982, p.347). The practitioner's sense of the physical body and self as identity (ego-identification) is obliterated, in order to 'commune' or 'form one body' with that which is outside of the self. For a speaker, this way of working with the breath has the potential to increase the connection with the listener. However, this ability develops through regular, long-term, rigorous practice and is not an ability readily available without training.

A third benefit of applying this way of breathing to Voice training is the cultivation of 'vocal presence' through the cultivation of ki. According to Lee there are three different kinds of ki in Korean. The first type, 'won-ki', is vital energy received from the mother in uterus via blood through the umbilical cord before breathing is possible. After birth, the blood of your parents is part of the won-ki energy you 'inherited'. To this, a second type, 'jong-ki', is now possible through breathing air via the lungs. Lee wrote, '(Jong-ki) is acquired energy from nourishment. The energy source is replenished through diet and respiration.' The third type, 'Jin-ki', is 'accessed through deep mindful concentration of the breath. . .Wherever in the body that you focus that is where the Jin-ki goes' (1999, p.33).

It is this third type of ki that I am interested in developing. This type of ki is 'a function which can not be perceived by ordinary consciousness in everyday life, but is a new function which consciousness (or mind) is gradually able to perceive through bodymind training in meditation and breathing methods' (Yuasa 1993, p.75–6).

The listener can perceive the 'consciousness' (or mind) of the performer and this perception contributes to a sense of the speaker's 'presence'. Presence can be understood through Barba's concept of 'pre-expressive' energy, which 'renders the (body/voice) theatrically "decided", "alive", . . . attracting the spectator's (listener's) attention before any form of message is transmitted' (www.odintheatret.dk/ista/anthropology.htm accessed 4 April 2008).

Adapting from Barba, pre-expressive energy can be understood as the foundation for the oral/aural exchange in training a speaker's voice and contributes to vocal presence because it readies not only the vocalist but the listener for what is to come. Both speaker and listener become present in what is being said and the speaker does this by learning how to shift one's ki as awareness, or consciousness, or 'mind' and harmonize with the listener. This process promotes more than effective oral/aural communication but a feeling of togetherness ('forming one body') that is a palpable, material condition of live performance.

DAHNJEON BREATHING EXERCISE

It is hoped that the above discussion helps better explain the objectives in training the breath/ki/mind embedded within this exercise. The exercise 'Dahnjeon Breathing' is a series of yoga asana positions which gradually 'wean' you from the floor to a standing position. Each asana uses the hardness of the floor, gravity, and the weight of your body to feel the breath/sound travel through your body, outside your body and across a distance to the listener. As you leave the floor into standing position, you must take responsibility for realizing the breath/sound production that gravity and the asana position was helping create moments before.

You must be attentive to the transitions between positions as well as live in each position itself. In this way, you can feel and hear how the architecture of the body shapes breath/sound production in motion and stillness, investigating the openness and closure of spaces in your body which effect breath/sound quality. Most importantly, as you embody the sequence, you must 'taste' (Oida and Marshall 1997, p.28) each asana position as you realize it through the growing integration of your bodymind.[5]

Below, the brief description of each asana position, directions for realizing the position, accompanied by a photo, addresses ki cultivation, bodymind integration as well as muscular contract/release cycles within the lower dahnjeon. However, for a western

---

5   The process of doing these exercises is similar to Yoshi Oida's understanding of 'tasting' the exercise. He wrote, 'When doing all these exercises, it is important to remind yourself to "taste" the movements. Doing them mechanically doesn't mean very much. You must try to notice the different sensations within the body' (1997, p.28).

readership the descriptions primarily address the skeletal-musculature. The directions refer to: spinal alignment for more efficient skeletal-muscular use, muscular contraction of the pelvic floor, transversus abdominis, internal obliques, (perhaps) external obliques and rectus abdominis depending on position and intensity of the muscular action. Also included in the directions are questions to provoke a learning response. Try your best to address each question with your bodymind, but do not expect an 'answer' or immediate result. You must commit to long-term, rigorous practice as you would with any training in order to begin realizing integrations of bodymind and ki cultivation and their beneficial effects on your breath/sound production.

First, breathe while realizing each position to discover how the body helps guide the breath as it travels through you, out of you and connects with the world around you. Then add simple counting, to the number ten perhaps, to hear how the efficiency of the skeletal-musculature is combining with ki. When you speak the words, 'one', 'two', 'three', etc. when counting, try to think of these words as simple vowel/consonant combinations that prepare you for more complex words. As you count you are feeling inside your body and listening to the sound in a rather technical way. Try working towards feeling and hearing a sense of 'strength' or support for the voice that seems 'effortless' or efficient. You are working technically to increase your awareness of the breath/sound and direct ki as 'awareness' as it travels through your body, out of your body and across a distance to a listener.

Finally, replace counting with a poem or other piece of text while realizing each position. This step introduces language and vocal expressiveness into your body/voice. Now you need to work towards combining technical proficiency with vocal expressiveness. When you live in each position or transition between positions notice how the body affects the voice, the sound and your ability to breath. Work towards feeling and hearing how the words emerge from your body. As the words emerge, try to link the feeling and sound of the words with the sense of what you are saying. Try to experience the experience of speaking, placing you in the here and now as you say each word, sentence, idea. Once you are standing speaking text at the end of the training sequence, continue speaking your text working towards feeling and hearing a 'strength' or focus and concentration of the sound within your speaking voice that effects intensity and quality and encourages the listener to involve themselves in what is being said. Work towards connecting with a listener and really communicating what you are saying.

EXERCISES[6]

Title: Dahnjeon breathing sequence

Aims: To train towards muscular efficiency in order to support the breath through the body, out of the body and across a distance to the listener. Through long-term, rigorous practice an additional aim is to create further levels of bodymind integration, cultivating ki (energy) which will give your sound a sense of strength beyond muscular strength and contribute to vocal presence in the here and now.

Where: A quiet, open space.

When: Daily if possible.

General notes

- In each position, match each inhalation with a muscular release and each exhalation with an efficient contraction. This intertwines each breath cycle with a muscular contract/release cycle. During each breathe cycle work towards realizing each asana position to discover how the body helps guide the breath as it travels through you, out of you, and connects with the world around you.

- Next, add simple counting, to the number ten perhaps, training towards listening and feeling the growing efficiency of the skeletal-musculature. When you speak the words, 'one', 'two', 'three', etc., try to think of these words as simple vowel/consonant combinations that prepare you for more complex words. As you count you are feeling inside your body and listening to the sound in a rather technical way.

- Now, count again only this time add an awareness of ki strength, working towards feeling and hearing a sense of strength or support for the voice that seems effortless or efficient beyond muscular efficiency.

- Finally, replace counting with a poem or other piece of text while realizing each position. This step introduces language and vocal expressiveness into your body/voice. The aim of this final step is to work towards combining technical proficiency with vocal expressiveness. When you live in each position or transition between positions notice how the body affects the voice, the sound and your ability to breathe. Work towards feeling and hearing how the words emerge

---

6   The position descriptions necessarily address the musculature for this chapter's intended western readership. Long-term, rigorous studio practice is essential for this kind of exercise and brief descriptions and photos cannot begin to articulate the phenomenological experience of ki-cultivation.

from your body. As the words emerge, try to link the feeling and sound of the words with the sense of what you are saying. Try to experience the experience of speaking, placing you in the here and now as you say each word, sentence, idea. Once you are standing speaking text at the end of the training sequence, continue speaking your text working towards feeling and hearing a 'strength' or focus and concentration of the sound within your speaking voice that effects intensity and quality and encourages the listener to involve themselves in what is being said. Work towards connecting with a listener and really communicating what you are saying.

- The overall structure of this sequence is an organized series of yoga asana positions which gradually 'wean' you from the floor to a standing position. Each asana uses the hardness of the floor, gravity and the weight of your body to feel the breath/sound travel through your body, outside your body and across a distance to the listener. As you leave the floor into standing position, you must take responsibility for realizing the breath/sound production that gravity and the asana position was helping create moments before.

- You must be attentive to the transitions between positions as well as live in each position itself. In this way, you can feel and hear how the architecture of the body shapes breath/sound production in motion and stillness, investigating the openness and closure of spaces in your body which effect breath/sound quality. Most importantly, as you embody the sequence, you must 'taste' (Oida and Marshall 1997, p.28) each asana position as you realize it through the growing integration of your bodymind.

- Below, the brief description of each asana position, directions for realizing the position, accompanied by a photo, addresses ki cultivation, bodymind integration as well as muscular contract/release cycles within the lower dahnjeon. However, for a western readership the descriptions primarily address the skeletal-musculature. The directions refer to: spinal alignment for more efficient skeletal-muscular use and muscular contraction of the pelvic floor, transversus abdominis, internal obliques, (perhaps) external obliques and rectus abdominis depending on position and intensity of the muscular action. Also included in the directions are questions to provoke a learning response. Try your best to address each question with your bodymind, but do not expect an 'answer' or immediate result. You must commit to long-term, rigorous practice as you would with any training in order to begin realizing integrations of bodymind and ki cultivation and their beneficial effects on your breath/sound production.

○ *Position One* A compliment to the 'Death' pose (*savasana*) in Hatha Yoga. To use the hardness of the floor, gravity and the weight of the body to feel the muscle groups of the lower dahnjeon during a contract/release cycle realized through resistance to the floor. To heighten your awareness of the relationship between the placement of the spine and the placement of the breath. (Note: Place your 'mind's eye,' or focused attention, into your back and notice how the slightest movement of the tailbone provides different forms of support to the lower dahnjeon.)

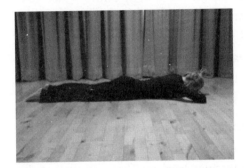 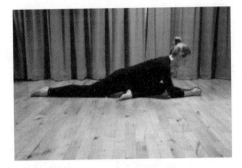

Figure 8.1   Figure 8.2

○ *Position Two* Leg Curls (right and left). With one leg at a time curled under the body on one side the aim is to increase the awareness of the working musculature during a full contract/release cycle. (Note: Allow the abdomen to rest on the thigh of the curled leg when in a released position. During the inhalation, notice how the musculature pushes against the curled leg. During the exhalation, can you feel the musculature contract away from the thigh? The feeling against the thigh helps you determine if you are accomplishing the full contract/release cycle within the abdomen).[7]

○ *Position Three* 'Half Lotus'.[8] To create awareness of a 'seat,' or triangle of support for the lower dahnjeon and a feeling of lifting the pelvic floor to support the voice through the body, out of the body, and across a distance to the listener. (Note: The 'seat' is comprised of three points – each buttock and the groin. You can feel the seat or pelvic floor release as it rests on the floor like a base for the spine. As the pelvic floor contracts it lifts slightly away from the floor. This contraction will help create the air pressure you need to travel

---

7   The author demonstrates the positions in Dahnjeon Breathing exercise. Photos by Roberto Ponzone, 2008.

8   In order to help you realize this position, try using an analogy that was explained to me by Bae Il-dong during one of my p'ansori lessons: the spine should be 'rooted' in this system of support like the roots of the lotus flower. The 'stalk' or spine 'grows' from the 'roots' (through alignment), with the head floating on the surface of the water like the lotus floats on a calm pond (lessons throughout 2003-4).

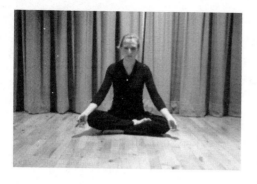

Figure 8.3

the breath/sound through the body, out of the body and across the distance to the listener. You will feel the muscles surrounding your anus engage during inhalation/exhalation and counting.[9]) A second aim is to help create further bodymind integration. (Note: Within this triangle of support floats the lower dahnjeon/ ki 'energy centre'. Place your mind's eye, or awareness, into the breath.

As you notice the breath come and go over a period of time you can let go of wilful management of the breath and breathing will seem effortless. The breath will have a sense of strength and firmness apart from muscular efficiency.)

○ *Position Four* The 'cat' position (*marjaravadivu*) adapted from my kalarippayattu training. Because this position lifts the pelvic floor off the studio floor, you now must take responsibility on a muscular level for the support that the studio floor, gravity and the weight of your body used to provide. (Note: This part of the 'weaning' process gives your body the opportunity to teach itself the muscular adjustments it needs to maintain muscular efficiency and still complete the task.) Focus your mind's eye on the placement of the spine and the placement of the breath in lower dahnjeon as you continue to notice the breath come and go.

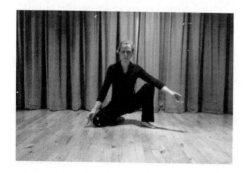

Figure 8.4

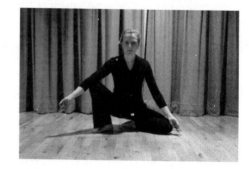

Figure 8.5

9   Refer to Oida and Marshall, 1997, p8–9. 'Even in performance, it [anus] isn't necessarily held clenched all the time. But at the most important moments, when the person needs to strike a powerful blow, or has to use the voice with great power, the anus is held tightly shut (8).'

○ *Position Five* 'Sitting'. This creates an awareness of the muscle groups on either side of the lower dahnjeon through the position of the thighs as support. (Note: Feel the breath as it is created in you, travels through you, travels out of you and meets with that which is outside of you. Try not to 'zone out', but create a connection with the world around you. Can you feel the space behind your back? On the top of your head? Shift your attention or awareness around your body, keeping yourself 'alive' in your developing bodymind.)

○ *Position Six* Kneeling – both knees on floor. By taking away the 'sitting' support, your body must teach itself how to adjust and take even more responsibility for supporting the lower dahnjeon muscles. (Note: This transition identifies if you are yet unable to tuck the tailbone beneath for support, or if you have a tendency to clench your abdomen muscles when righting yourself in a semi-standing position. Or, in this position you might be tempted to increase the natural curvature of the lower spine, collapsing into your body instead of building the spine as a means of support. Take a moment to notice how your body shifts the support and takes responsibility for this task. What part of your musculature can you let go of and still accomplish this simple task? How efficient can your use of the skeletal-musculature become in simply transitioning from 'sitting' into 'kneeling'? Where is your awareness as you accomplish this task?)

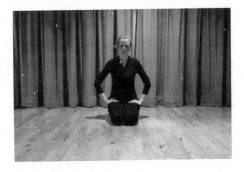

Figure 8.6

○ *Position Seven* Right and left leg. Kneeling – one knee on floor. This position increases an awareness of the muscles on either side of the lower dahnjeon by providing contrasting support during one-knee kneeling. (Note: Place your awareness in the spine as if it were still rooted to the floor. Your kneeling leg will help you feel this connection between the floor and the lower dahnjeon. Even as your body begins to stand upright, continue to feel this link with the floor.)

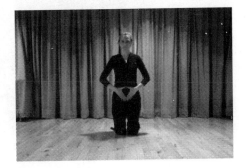

Figure 8.7

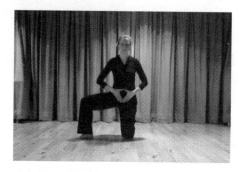

Figure 8.8

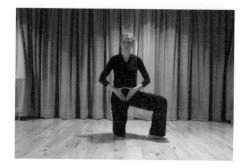

Figure 8.9

- ○ *Position Eight* Patsy Rodenburg's 'kabuki' position (Rodenburg, *A Voice of Your Own* [DVD]). This position encourages the appropriate position for the spine as it affects the tilt of the pelvic floor, helping to support the voice through the body, out of the body and across a distance to the listener. (Note: Imagine you are about to sit on a tall stool, putting your awareness in the spine as if it is rooted to the floor. Focus your attention, or awareness, on the relationship between the placement of the spine and the placement of the breath in lower dahnjeon.) Another aim is to feel muscular and ki awareness in this position. (Note: Place your awareness behind you, above you, in front of you. Feel ki extend through the soles of your feet into the floor and from the top of your head simultaneously. Strive towards that feeling of being present in this time and in this place, connecting to the world around you as you notice the breath come and go.)

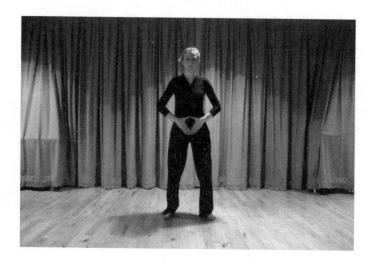

Figure 8.10

○ *Position Nine* Left and right legs. The 'horse' position (*asvavadivu*) adapted from my kalarippayattu training. This position's aim is to feel the ki extend from the top of your head and through the soles of your feet simultaneously. (Note: In this position, you may be particularly tempted to bend your spine so that your chin tilts up and eyes are looking at the wall in front of you. However, you should align the spine, which will bring your external eye looking at the floor a bit away from your position. You should continue to put your mind's eye or internal eye into your spine, creating a relationship with the placement of the spine and the placement of the breath in lower dahnjeon.)

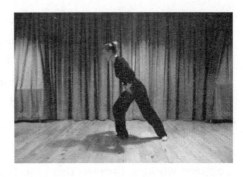

Figure 8.11

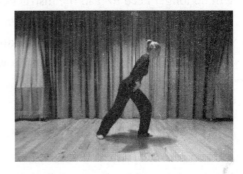

Figure 8.12

○ *Position Ten* Left and right legs – the 'crane'. This position cultivates the feeling of a full contract/release cycle as gravity helps the lower dahnjeon muscles to release towards the floor and cultivate the feeling of ki as it circulate around your bodymind. Can you feel ki extend off the top of your head and out through the soles of your feet simultaneously? Can you place your awareness behind you?

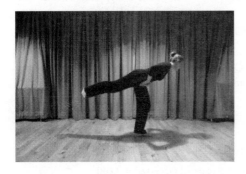

Figure 8.13

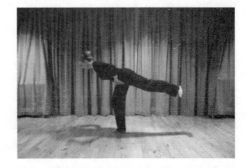

Figure 8.14

○ *Position Eleven* Standing. This position integrates muscular efficiency with ki strength during speaking. Also, to create a sense of speaking that connects with the world around you in the here and now. Can you feel inside your body a sense of ease as you support the breath/sound through your body, out of your body and across a distance to a listener? Can you hear a focused energy in your sound, perhaps giving your sound a 'strength' or purpose or direction?

Continue working through this sequence with any text you are preparing for a listener. With regular practice your bodymind will remember the sequence and you will no longer need to read the instructions from this paper. As you work, remember 'voice is acoustic reflection of mind' (Park 2003, p.189). As the voice moves so the mind moves and as the mind moves so does the voice. One does not follow the other but both are together in the here and now, absorbed with the listener in the moment of speaking/listening.

BIBLIOGRAPHY

Barba, Eugenio and Savarese, Nicola (1991) *A Dictionary of Theatre Anthropology*. London: Routledge.

Benedetti, Robert (1990) *The Actor at Work*. New Jersey: Prentice Hall.

Kasulis, Thomas P. with Ames, Roger T. and Dissanayake, Wimal (eds) (1993) *Self as Body in Asian Theory and Practice*. Albany: State University of New York Press.

Leder, Drew (1990) *The Absent Body*. Chicago: University of Chicago Press.

Lee, Seung-Heun (1999) *Dahnhak*. Seoul: Dahn Publications.

Nearman, Mark (1982) 'Kakyo: A Mirror of the Flower. Part One.' *Monumenta Nipponica 37*, 3 343–74.

Oida, Yoshi and Marshall, Lorna, (1997) *The Invisible Actor*. London: Methuen.

Park, Chan E. (2003) *Voices from the Straw Mat: Toward Ethnography of Korean Story Singing*. Honolulu: University of Hawaii Press.

Rodenburg, Patsy (2005) *A Voice of Your Own* (DVD). New York/London: Applause Theatre and Cinema Books.

Um, Hae-Kyung (1992) *Making P'ansori: Korean Musical Drama*. The Queen's University of Belfast: Unpublished PhD: Ethnomusicology.

Yoo, Jeungsook. (2007) 'Moving Ki in Inner and Outer Space: A Korean Perspective on Acting Process in The Water Station', *Contemporary Theatre Review 17*, 1, 81–96.

Websites

www.odintheatret.dk/ista/anthropology.htm (accessed 4.4.08)

http://www.youtube.com/results?search_query=pansori&page=2 (accessed 4.4.08)

CHAPTER 9

Transformative Breath

From Shamanism to voice practice

MARJ MCDAID

In a brief yet powerful contact with a movement practitioner named Nelly Dougar-Zhabon at the CPR Archaeology of the Voice conference in Aberystwyth in 1997 a new and exciting dimension was added to my voice teaching practice. Dougar-Zhabon, originally a movement teacher at the Eastern Siberian Institute of Culture in Ulan-Ude, spent a period of eight years under the guidance of a shaman, and developed a training based on her experiences, which integrates vocal and physical training and enables performers to develop and sustain inner voice energies, emotional flexibility, physical and plastic expression. The core of this training is a series of exercises combining breath and movement. In my work with students I have come to use these regularly, and they soon came to be known as the Shamans – a term I shall use throughout this chapter.

Sadly, Dougar-Zhabon died shortly after our initial meeting before the full scope of her work could be communicated to a wider audience. I have subsequently sought to deepen my understanding of the practice she imparted and in this chapter I will examine the various influences which inspired her work, principally the nature of Siberian shamanism, but also Tibetan Dynamic Meditation and Chi Gong.

I shall draw links with approaches to performance breath for vocal communication, of which I have experiential and theoretical knowledge and with which Dougar-Zhabon's work resonates, the work of Rudolf Laban, Stanislav Grof's holotropic breath work, Alfred Wolfsohn, and, minimally but significantly, the ideas of Deepak Chopra. What all these share is the significance of the emotional power of the breath. I shall also use the insights and terminology of Jo Estill's Voicecraft to describe the exercises.

SHAMANISM: AN OVERVIEW

First, then: shamanism itself. The central function of a shaman is to act as an intermediary between the people of a community and the spirit world, in order to strengthen and sustain community and bring healing. In order to do so, he or she enters into a trance-like state, an altered state of consciousness. Over-breathing may be a small part of achieving that state, as may fasting, but the principal method used in Siberia is fast drumming. In shamanism in other parts of the world, psychotropic plant extracts are the usual way of reaching such states. In Siberia the Amanita muscaria mushroom is used, albeit rarely. Dougar-Zhabon must have recognized that actors' performances could be lifted to another level were they to achieve the intensity of performance usual in shamanistic practice. However, her physiological approach was to make breathing, rather than drumming or drugs, central to the process and to incorporate Tibetan Dynamic Meditation. This is why I believe this work is so effective in my teaching and why it has a rightful place in this collection.

Prior to my investigations, I had the idea that a shaman was an older person in the community, who was sought for their wisdom and healing. I was surprised to learn that shamans are selected when they are young and are trained. They are frequently chosen because of some kind of sickness, which usually has a psychological dimension, hence their being referred to as 'the wounded healer' or 'the healed teacher' (Thorpe 1993, p. 38). There does not appear to be etymological agreement about the origins of the word 'shaman' but one suggestion is that it may be from the Manchu word 'Saman' – one who is excited, moved or raised (Thorpe 1993, ch.2). The historian Ronald Hutton, in *Shamans: Siberian Spirituality and the Western Imagination*, says that if shamanism was partly craft and partly a spiritual vocation it was also an aspect of theatre and often a spectacularly effective one (2001, p. 85). The ethnologist Vilmos Dioszegi, in *Tracing Shamans in Siberia*, may have felt that all the shamans he met were misfits, but he also credited each with exceptional skill as a performer: one was a great singer, another an expressive dancer, one had exceptional dramatic skills, another was an evocative raconteur and so on (Hutton 2001, p. 86).

The novelist and anthropologist Waclaw Sieroszewski wrote of shamans,

> for some of them dispose of light and darkness in such a masterly manner, but also of silence and incantation – the modulation of the voice is so flexible, the gestures so peculiar and expressive … that involuntarily you give yourself into the charm of watching this wild and free evocation of a wild and free spirit. (Hutton 2001, p. 86)

Another description – this time of a shamaness – from Dioszegi is worth noting.

> The voice of the shamaness had not become louder, she did not raise it at all, her recitation did not become faster. And in spite of that, the atmosphere was filled with tension' (Hutton 2001, p. 278). On another occasion, under the influence of the shaman's song, 'the little ones forgot to cry, they let go of the nipples and they listened, too' (ibid.).

In the academic studies of shamanism there seems to be consensus that a central part of shamanistic practice is role taking. In social psychology, of course, there is a huge body of knowledge called Role Theory, which interprets all of our social behaviour in terms of the roles we play in everyday life. Considering shamanism in the light of role theory from a psycho-sociological point of view, Sarbin and Allen, in their analysis of a role performance, identify that there is a triad: (1) the role performer, (2) the person in the complementary role and (3) a third member who observes the process of social interaction (or, in other words, the audience) and draws the conclusion that 'it is of primary importance to examine not the only the shaman's behaviour but also his relationship towards his audience' (Siikala 1978, p. 61). In social situations role taking is usually short and superficial but in some cases it can go much deeper. Sarbin studied the changes in psycho-physical states in role taking, observing people under hypnotism and the work of the actor. He concluded that when role taking becomes deeply identified with the other it might lead to role change. Role taking depends on previous experience. With role change the individual enters into the very consciousness of the other. So the shaman, in order to mediate between this and the spirit world, as it were becomes the spirit. It is obvious that the central part of the actor's work is to take on roles. The aspiration of the actor is to totally inhabit the character. The parallels with shamanic practice are clear. But with role-play having become an integral part of many in-service training programmes, where the importance of communication has been recognized, then the relevance goes way beyond the stage.

The main duty of the shaman is the maintenance of clan coherence. He does this by role changing – i.e. embodying the Spirit. In so doing, the shaman uplifts the individual out of the harsh realities of existence and at the same time makes individuals more connected to each other. Likewise in the western world, where material conditions are much more comfortable but where the sense of community is weaker than in primitive societies, one of the roles of the performer – if not the key role, even in light entertainment – is to overcome existential loneliness, disconnectedness. If society benefits in this passive way, how much more benefit may derive from engaging actively in processes such as the shamanic exercises which will be described later.

TRANSFORMATION IN SHAMANISM AND PERFORMANCE

The most profound challenge for the good actor is the ability to transform – the dancer likewise, in the context of ballet, classical or contemporary. With singers too, when they really inhabit the music and the lyrics, they transform. The act of singing affects the body's chemistry: we can feel high, connected to the universe, somehow larger than our normal selves. Looking at transformation in communities where shamanism is still practised, the cosmologist A.F. Anisimov, in *Cosmological Concepts of the Peoples of the North*, gives an example of narrative turning into a perpetual motion of forms in mythological transformations, 'a girl, in hiding from the moon, changes into a hillock, a lamp, a stone block, a hammer, a pole, a sack, a particle of the Earth – even a short hair on the hide of the bed curtains' (1963, p. 217). What an inspiration for theatre!

Anisimov explains that, 'in the view of the Chukchi (tribe) such transformations appeared possible because they supposed nature was endowed with life and its transfer from one state to another constituted a natural phenomenon of this general creativity of life' (1963, p. 217). Every material object and animal 'has its own voice'. With this view of the world real transformation is much more viable than in the western worldview. Nevertheless, transformation is still the aspiration of the performer. When it is achieved the audience is taken into another world. The majority of people may not have transformation as a priority goal, but many people do want to live in a more vital, authentic manner.

LABAN LINKS

In addition to the obvious links to Shaman traditions found in Dougar-Zhabon's work, links to more modern and widely known performance practices can be found. In the work of Rudolf Laban (see Chapter 16 by Katya Bloom), his core views on movement, established from observing people working in industry, are based on the belief that movement is the result of a state of mind or striving after an object deemed valuable (von Laban 1960, p. 87). Its shapes and rhythms show the moving person's attitude in a particular situation. It can characterize momentary mood and reactions as well as more constant features of personality. The bodily attitudes during movement are determined by two main action forms: one flowing from the periphery of the space surrounding the body to the centre – 'gathering'; the other flowing from the centre of the body outwards – 'scattering'. These features are notable in Dougar-Zhabon's exercises.

Laban's belief that theatre transcends ordinary everyday experiences resonates strongly with the shamanistic experience, as does his view of the magnetic current running between the poles of the happenings on stage and the audience.

Many readers will be familiar with Laban's categorization of movements in which he analyses the fundamental movements that can be applied to the expression of inner states of mind and emotions in terms of tempo, weight and direction. These characteristics are also very evident in the Shamans, but with the focus being on the breath.

THE HOLOTROPIC BREATH WORK CONNECTION

In the world of performance and throughout holistic practice the connection between breath and the emotions is well recognized, explored and written about. The most extreme experience I myself have had of the connection between breath and the psyche was on a holotropic breath workshop. It is certainly the closest I have got to the shamanistic experience. Holotropic breath work was developed by Stanislav Grof and his wife Christina. Grof is a psychiatrist who has researched into non-ordinary states of consciousness. These were induced originally by psychedelic substances but when these were banned he was able to replicate them by other means, principally over-breathing. I find this fascinating because Dougar-Zhabon, following a non-scientific path, has done essentially the same thing.

I attended a holotropic breath workshop because of my fascination with the psycho-physical aspect of breathing, but with very little knowledge of what to expect. I did my three hours breathing with a 'sitter' in charge, in a large room with about

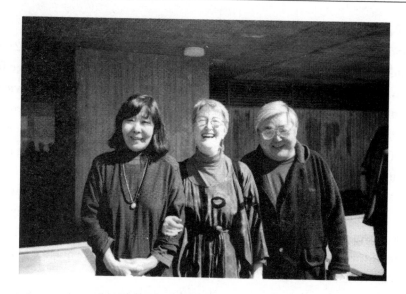

Figure 9.1 Nelly Dougar-Zhabon, Mar, McDaid and Nelly's husband Bair

seventy other breathers and sitters (we took it in turn to 'sit' and to breathe). There was music playing throughout. I met none of my old psychological demons. In fact the opposite happened. I had the most blissful experience of God who took the form of a horse – not a realistic horse, more like an animated wire construction of a horse! And of the deep, gentle caring nature of God. It was literally extra-ordinary. Moreover, I remained in a buoyant peacefulness for a long time – several months. I recount this story because it is a direct experience of the power of breath and I went into this altered state of consciousness with no preconceived ideas about such a possibility. The medical profession regards hyperventilation as pathological. In rare circumstances it is induced, for example in the case of brain injury, in order to reduce the pressure on the brain, but in most cases it would be 'treated' in order to stop it or prevent it. Grof, however, holds that when people hyperventilate spontaneously it is the body/mind's way of attempting to self-heal (Grof 1990, p. 90). And certainly the induced hyperventilation, for me, was wonderfully positive.

LINKS WITH OTHER EASTERN DISCIPLINES

Much of my thought and research has centred on shamanism because Dougar-Zhabon was a native of Siberia which, along with inner Asia, is described by the anthropologist Anna-Leena Siikala as the *locus classicus* for shamanism (1978). It was Dougar-Zhabon's culture and it undoubtedly had a huge influence on her, even before she put herself under the guidance of a particular shaman. Tibetan Dynamic Meditation

(TDM), the other major influence acknowledged by Dougar-Zhabon, needs less exposition because its philosophy and practice are more familiar territory. Its purpose is the spiritual development of the body's major energy channels. The focus of the movement is the chakras, the crossing-points of these channels. Precise fluid movements shift the focus from one chakra to another in a gentle manner. In the Shamans a stronger energy is used, but the idea of concentrating and shifting the energy is integral to them and is observable.

Although Dougar-Zhabon made no direct reference to the Chinese discipline of Chi-Gong, there are several facets of this discipline that facilitate an understanding of her exercises. The Chi-Gong master directs and manipulates energy to transmit it to his students, allowing them to raise their level of energy. The exercises, combined with the teacher's presence and intention to transmit energy, cause this to happen. This is a model for how the Shamans are conducted. The should be done with a teacher until they are thoroughly internalized.

Gunnel Minett, an organizational psychologist and rebirthing practitioner/researcher, in her overview of how breathing is used throughout the world, describes the Chinese view which divides the effects of breathing into three categories: effects on the body, the psyche and the spirit (1994, pp. 37–41). The variables that produce these effects are variations in speed of breathing, the depth of each breath and the length of each breath. She found scientific studies of Chi-Gong practice which appear to have established that several natural, physical emissions from the body, such as infra-red radiation, static electricity and various particle radiations are all affected in a measurable way by the practice of breathing according to Chi-Gong methods (Minett 1994, p. 38). This system for codifying types of breath and their effects on the body/mind is strongly reflected in Dougar-Zhabon's work.

THE SIGNIFICANCE OF ATTENTION AND INTENTION

In the course of writing this chapter there has been a growing awareness about the respective roles of intention and attention in breathing. It struck me that when teaching voice or singing, the teacher is constantly modelling breathing for the students or simply doing it along with them, but we are not affected by that breathing in the same way as the student. This must be because our attention is on the student. Our intention is to facilitate and be observant of the student. If we were to go back into the role of student, for example in attending a workshop, then we would be affected differently by the same type of breathing. My conclusion is that while the breath is an amazingly subtle yet powerful vehicle or transmitter, it is dependent on both intention and attention. Stanislav Grof's findings would seem to support this view: 'an element that is essential in Holotropic therapy or self-exploration – sustained, focused introspection' (2000, p. 185).

Paradoxically, one of the many reasons that we work on breathing with our students is to increase focused attention. If we are following the path of the breath in the body we are literally becoming more aware of ourselves. But if we breathe, however deeply, without that attention, does it have the same effect? I suspect not. I think it has some effect, but not as profound. So the actual physical breath, of itself, would seem not to be the transformer. It would seem to be dependent upon intention and attention.

The relevance of attention is further supported by the work of Deepak Chopra, the endocrinologist who went back to his Indian roots and the use of Ayurvedic medicine and has been a significant bridge-builder between western science and eastern mysticism. In making the case for the power of meditation he draws on the developments in quantum physics. He asserts that when our attention is not on particles, they are just a mathematical probability, because a particle is a wave at the same time. It is a wave until the moment of observation. A wave is not restricted to any one location in space and time. A wave defines the statistical likelihood of finding a particle at a certain place at the time of observation. It is attention that transforms that 'probability amplitude' and brings it into material existence, 'so a particle is literally created by you and me through the act of observation' (Chopra 1993). Again, as Grof says, 'consciousness does not just passively reflect the objective material world: it plays an active role in creating reality itself' (1990, p. 10).

The Shamans can be done, as it were, 'in neutral', simply to shift the energies and to feel the effect of this on the voice. The extent of their transformative power is affected by the attention with which they are performed. And when they are done in preparation for a performance they are informed by the work the performer has done on the intentions and actions of the character or song. Likewise, a business person preparing for a presentation would bring a specific set of intentions, which would inform the exercises. The embodiment of these intentions then changes the experiences of the Shamans. So the same exercises have a quite different psychological feeling to them depending on the intention inherent in a particular context and the attention with which they are performed.

THE END OF THE BREATH

To breathe in order to achieve a state of calm is widely recognized – 'take a deep breath' is a common admonition. Dougar-Zhabon has taken this common insight to its logical conclusion by developing this set of exercises: twelve different ways of breathing that lead into different emotional energies. In the Shamans the breath is shaped and reshaped. Sometimes it is like a deep, slow-moving river; sometimes like a fast-moving stream. This reshaping throughout the twelve exercises is in response to changes in physicality – facial expression and body movement – which also suggest an attitude. We may 'take a deep' breath to become calmer, but who thinks to breathe in a different way in order to become more energetic? Or, indeed, to have a more compelling effect such as a politician might wish to achieve.

In a number of the Shamans the breath is held to the very last drop. There seems to be support by experts in the field as to the beneficial effects of going to the very end of the breath. Kristin Linklater's exercise of 'vacuuming the lungs' is an example (1976, pp. 126–8).

Going to the very end of the breath was also used by Alfred Wolfsohn but in his case using the voice on a single pitch as well. Wolfsohn, best known through the Roy Hart theatre in France, was interested in taking the voice to its highest and lowest, into the cracks of the voice and by that means penetrating the psyche. In my own experience of doing this work with Derek Gale, who has carried on Wolfsohn's work in England, I found that this mainly came about in myself and others through the intensity of going to the last drop of breath.

In the Shamans, going to the very end of the breath happens most strongly in number three but it also occurs in two, six and seven and probably accounts in part for their transformative effect. The repetition on the following breaths without any gaps also minimizes the possibility of resistance occurring.

THE EXERCISES

Unlike a lot of voice work, the Shamans are conducted in rows, in chess formation, so that everyone can have eye contact with the leader. The students mimic the leader. The leader, as it were, gives the energy to the group, following the model of the shaman's practice. Using the Shamans is a wonderful way to focus and to ground a group. They can also be used with individuals.

Each of the 12 exercises is repeated four times. This is both to internalize it and to instil a sense of discipline. They combine physical movement with an inhalation and an exhalation. Most represent approximate character types or attitudes, using different speeds of inhalation and exhalation, different laryngeal postures, different strengths, different tempi. The out-breath is on a specified vowel, all except two being unvoiced. Two are about maintaining energized calm, for example, before performance or undertaking an onerous task, and one is about generosity towards the audience and receptivity to the audience's energy as well as evoking a particular voice quality. The particular voice quality is set up on the in-breath, which is always through the nose. For example in number three there is a strong, noisy pulling in of the breath with the nostrils becoming really distended, whereas in number two the nostrils remain soft and there is no sound.

The exercises take us through a range of energies and qualities, all on the breath. Each one is followed by a voiced count of eight in the quality already experienced in the vocal mechanism during the out-breath. Each exercise can then be repeated, followed by an excerpt of text instead of the count of eight.

Dougar-Zhabon was adamant that her work was part of an ongoing oral tradition, so the exercises do not exist in a written or diagrammatic form. I feel privileged to be part of that tradition and out of respect for it will just describe the exercises sufficiently to convey how they work. I believe the most accurate way of conveying them is to describe them in terms of Jo Estill's system, Voicecraft, as this is a system recognized world-wide (a summary of the Estill method is presented in the appendix). All are executed with a strong laugh position in the throat (Estill's deconstriction). Voice use can be either speech or singing.

Table 9.1 'The Shamans' described making use of Estill's terminology

	Type	Vowel	Voice use	Tempo
1	Practical, direct	Whispered (aː)	Thick folds, medium larynx, medium pitch	Medium, sustained, cut off
2	Light, smooth	Silent (a)	Thin folds, medium larynx, medium to high pitch	Slower, sustained
3	Very strong, bold	Whispered (æ)	Thick folds, low larynx, wide pharynx, twang, low pitch	Very slow, sustained
4	Youthful, bright	Whispered (hæ)	Thick folds, medium to high larynx, wide pharynx, medium to high pitch	Medium to fast, sudden

Table 9.1 *cont.*

	Type	Vowel	Voice use	Tempo
5	Bimbo, silly person	Voiced (hi:)–(hi:)	High larynx, thin folds, twang, high pitch	Quite fast, shaken out
6	Sensuous	Whispered (ɔ:)	Low larynx, thin folds, low pitch	Slow, sustained
7	Raunchy	Voiced (ɔ:)	Low larynx, thick folds, low pitch	Faster than 6, shaken out
8	Mean, sharp	Voiced French "u"	Very high larynx, thick folds, lot of twang, medium to high pitch	Ad lib
9	Speedy, direct	Unvoiced (hæ)	Medium larynx, thick folds, twang	Very fast, staccato
10	Generous, warm	Unvoiced (a:)	Low larynx, wide pharynx, thick or thin folds	Slow, sustained

The final two exercises are about keeping both relaxed and energized before a performance, public speaking or presentations and are not used to produce specific voice qualities. In number 11 the hands are clenched and unclenched rapidly while inhaling and exhaling four times. In number 12, again while breathing in and out four times, the backs of the hands are massaged with the fingertips and a hand-washing movement is used. In both, the heels are raised on the in-breath and lowered to the ground on the out-breath.

Examples of the movements used in numbers 3 and 9 are given in the practice section at the end.

APPLICATION IN THE DRAMA TRAINING ENVIRONMENT

How do I use the Shamans in the context of drama school training? Dougar-Zhabon made it clear that they were not a substitute for skills training, and that in fact they work most effectively with people who already have a sound and movement, voice and acting training. So I made the decision not to introduce them until near the end of the second term of the second year in a three-year training course. I leave explanations until after I have done them, allowing the students to make their own discoveries about them. Many students take to them instantly, a few are initially resistant and some just think I am a bit wacky! All at first think they are quite hilarious, as I did myself when I first did them with Nelly herself.

I use them in class on a regular basis, getting the students moving in the manner of the exercise as well as speaking. Dougar-Zhabon used to talk about 'all the little people we have inside us'. We can give expression to these in the format of the exercises. When the students are working towards a production, once they have had time to explore their characters I suggest they create their own character-specific exercise: that is, one that expresses the character's typical modus operandi. This encourages them to trust the work they have done, to let go of thinking, to find their character's voice intuitively and to express that psycho-physically. This can happen both in class and in a tutorial situation.

Having used them during the rehearsal process, I then use them as warm-ups before performance. In this way the actors are quickly shifted from one quality to another, from one energy to another. A character may have a predominant disposition. The good actor will not play that one state, but be responsive, moment-to-moment, with the shifting wants and actions of the character. It seems to me that the Shamans reinforce this facility.

They are most obviously useful in works which require extreme vocal qualities: when I recently coached on Mervyn Peakes's Gormenghast they were indispensable. But in fact they are equally effective for more subtle voice use. This is clear from the following extracts from my students' logbooks:

> *Laura*: 'We began exploring vocal characterization and access to character through breath and physicality today using the Shamans. These instantly engage your body and your breath to a specific state, emotion or type of person and additionally can be many aspects of one individual character.'

> *Bethan*: 'I found that this was the most helpful thing we did all term and actually, this was my key to finding a grounded voice for Portia and Solanio.' She found numbers 1 and 8 helpful: 'This brought up a more grounded, resonant quality to my voice, which the director had been striving to get. I felt particularly rooted and felt that I was bringing the words from my guts. This was an absolute breakthrough for me as it gave me a way into the voice quality and, if I felt in danger of losing it at any point, I could revert back to the Shaman. No. 8 was useful (but not as useful!) for Solanio. It is similar to no. 1 but much quicker. I found the quicker exhalations led me to a more boyish, boisterous quality.'

Dan: 'The Shamans help you to explore different states of energy and also affect the tone and texture of your voice. They help to stimulate new and creative ways of bringing a character to life.'

Jonny: 'I found the Shamans brought fluidity to the character, which connected numerous qualities of the character without too much intellectual thought, bringing a different energy without too much effort. I could achieve a lot with relative ease and this allowed me to remain free and at ease as a person.'

As I have indicated throughout, I see the Shamans' usefulness extending beyond the actor to the general workplace. I am also convinced that they would be very effective psychotherapeutically – an area still to be explored. My initial impulse to research and subsequently write came from a desire to bring Nelly Dougar-Zhabon's work to a larger audience. The process has brought me closer to understanding not only why the work is so effective but also how and why breath work can be so powerful. Shamanism shares with other eastern schools of thought a view of reality in which mind and spirit are one. The breath techniques are used to shift the awareness from the rational to the intuitive mode of consciousness. Nelly alerted me to the fact that intuition is not a substitute for intellectual learning nor for the acquisition of skills. Intuition is immediate insight, bypassing the reasoning process but using all accumulated knowledge – intellectual, physical, emotional, which is exactly what any performer needs.

The Shamans, when you know them, only take about ten minutes to do, but they are the product of a vibrant, rich tradition and consequently touch us at many levels. I use them as part of the actor's development and as part of the preparation for a performance because, as well as going through a range of vocal qualities and energies, they focus and unite the players and bring them into intuitive mode. I also use them with people outside the theatrical world who are seeking to develop vocally. They encapsulate the core elements of those approaches to voice work that have most profoundly influenced me – from the precise mechanical system of Jo Estill, through Linklater, Laban's Directions, to Wolfsohn's connection of the raw voice to the psyche. And they do this through the medium of the breath, which connects to my own core belief in the Spirit.

EXERCISES

Title: Change of Expression

Aim: To experience how changing your expression can alter the manner of breathing.

Experiment with two contrasting facial expressions and experience how you breathe differently. For example:

- Raise one eyebrow, harden your eyes, sneer with closed lips.

- Breathe in through the nostrils, breathe out through an open mouth, keeping the sneer.

- Now soften the eyes, gently smile, incline the head to one side.

- Breathe in through the nostrils, exhale through an open mouth, keeping the smile.

Was there a change in the way the breath was taken in? – its speed, strength, sound? Likewise on the out-breath.

Title: Sweet Sustained (*Shaman* no. 2)

Aim: To achieve a smooth, pleasant manner of speaking.

- Stand with feet shoulders' width apart.

- Extend arms level with shoulders.

- Bring thumb and forefinger together on each hand.

- With soft eyes, slight smile, breathe in silently through nostrils while bringing the hands gracefully, moderately slowly, towards the mouth, and at the same time going on to the ball of the foot.

- Release the breath silently with smiling mouth shaped in an 'ah', extending the arms again gracefully and returning heels to floor.

- This is all done with a feeling of generosity.

- Do this four times.

- Immediately do a spoken count to eight, keeping the same space in the vocal tract and the same slow pace of the preceding movements.

- Do the movements again four times and then speak some text in the same manner.

Title: Fast Thrust (*Shaman* no. 9)

Aim: To move into rapid, direct delivery of speech.

- Stand with feet a shoulders' width apart.

- Place hands on waist, thumbs forward.

- On the in-breath through the nostrils, do a fast swipe down the back of the legs while dropping the head towards the feet.

- Extremely quickly, come upright, hands back on waist.

- With lips spread wide and a strong laugh position in the throat, exhale on a short, staccato 'A' (as in 'cat') with a fast thrust forward of the pelvis (sound like an angry cat!).

- Do this four times very fast.

- Immediately do a spoken count to eight, without the movements, keeping the same space in the vocal tract and the same fast pace of the preceding movements.

- Repeat the movements again four times.

- Speak the same piece of text again in the same manner.

Experience the difference in the voice qualities, the different attitudes, the different energy between nos. 2 and 3.

APPENDIX

Jo Estill's system is a mechanistic approach to voice training for both speech and singing developed from laboratory observations of the physiology of the vocal mechanism – the larynx and vocal tract. The premise is that the structures can be independently controlled, thus altering the vocal quality. For simplicity's sake, for my purposes here I shall focus on the basic structures and their acoustic consequences, only elucidating terms needed to describe Nelly's exercises.

- The false folds can constrict or retract. When constricted they interfere with the free vibration of the true folds. The retracted position therefore is recommended for healthy vocalisation. This is achieved by a strong "laugh" position in the throat.

- The larynx can move up and down. Usually it rests in the middle position. A high larynx position creates a thinner, clearer, brighter tone; a low larynx position results in a fuller tone.

- The vocal folds can be adjusted to be either thick or thin. Thick folds produce the quality usually described as "chest voice" – strong, with a slight edge to the sound. Thin fold quality is usually described as "head voice" – softer, sweeter in tone.

- The pharynx can be widened, again producing a fuller sound because of the increased space.

- The soft palate can be raised or lowered. When completely lowered to meet the raised tongue the sound is nasal. When partially lowered there can be degrees of nasality.

- The top of the trachea can be tightened forming the aryepiglottic sphincter, renamed by Jo "the twanger" because the sound produced when it is tightened is like the twang of a guitar. The sound is very bright and penetrating. It can be nasal, but its most useful application is when it is oral.

By using a "recipe" of different combinations of the structures, countless voice qualities are produced. In Voicecraft, Estill did not deal with breath. She recognised that there were other aspects to voice – artistry and "magic" or the metaphysics of performance. In Nelly's work we get some of the latter as well as incorporating the physiological techniques.

BIBLIOGRAPHY

Anisimov, A.F. (1963) *Cosmological Concepts of the Peoples of the North.* Ed. Henry N. Michael. *Studies in Siberian Shamanism.* Arctic Institute of N. America: University of Toronto Press.

Chopra, Deepak (1993) *Creating Affluence* (Audiocassette). Novato: Amber-Allan New World Library.

Grof, Stanislav (1990) *The Holotropic Mind.* San Francisco: Harper.

Grof, Stanislav (2000) *Psychology of the Future.* New York: State University of New York Press.

Hutton, Ronald (2001) *Shamans: Siberian Spirituality and the Western Imagination.* London: Hambledon.

Linklater, Kristin (1976) *Freeing the Natural Voice.* New York: Drama Book Publishers.

Minett, Gunnel (1994) *Breath and Spirit.* London: HarperCollins.

Thorpe, S.A. (1993) *Shamans, Medicine Men and Traditional Healers.* Koedoespoort: University of SA Pretoria.

Saint-Denis, Michel (1982) *Training for the Theatre: Premises and Promises.* Ed. Suria Saint-Denis. New York: Theatre Art Books.

Siikala, Anna-Leena (1978) *The Rite Technique of the Siberian Shaman.* Helsinki: Folklore Fellows Communications.

von Laban, Rudolf (1960) *The Mastery of Movement: 2nd Edition.* Ed. Lisa Ullman. Boston: Plays.

CHAPTER 10

Qi Gong Breathing[1]

MICHAEL MORGAN

INTRODUCTION

Qi (pronounced 'chee') is the energy extracted from air through breathing and *gong* refers to the practice of physical and mental movements that facilitate this process. While standard definitions of *qi gong* leave no doubt about the centrality of the breath, since the phrase is typically translated from the Chinese as breathing (*qi*) work (*gong*), it must be acknowledged that the concept of *qi* is complex. It often is associated with the Hindu term *prana* (the breath of life). *Qi* is most commonly translated as energy. This is because there is something that both terms, *qi* and energy, share in their universal application as vitalizing power or life force.

In approaching the subject of *qi gong* breathing, it will be useful to briefly introduce the undergirding terminology of Taoist esoteric anatomy that informs this practice. According to Taoist thought – influenced by Traditional Chinese Medicine – the human body houses a trio of substances: *jing, qi* and *shen*, known as the three treasures. There are two kinds of *jing*: congenital and acquired.

Congenital *jing* is the fundamental essence of the physical body contributed by the parents at the time of conception and is, therefore, inherited. It governs overall constitution, growth and development and corresponds to the contemporary concept of DNA. Pre-natal *jing* is seen as a precious, irreplaceable treasure that is stored in the

---

1   The illustrations are by Brittany Howard.

Kidneys. Because *jing* governs life cycles from infancy to old age, its preservation is very significant to the practice of *qi gong* that aims at increasing longevity.

After birth, *jing* is extracted from food. The Spleen, considered the organ of digestion, controls acquired or post-natal *jing*, the essence that replenishes vitality. Both pre and post-natal *jing* are favourably influenced by the health-seeking breathing practices of *qi gong*.

Shen is similar to the concept of spirit in western terminology and is also called mind. As such, it has a particular connation as human consciousness. *Shen*'s chief residence is the Heart, but *shen*, generated at the navel during the time of birth, also spreads through the organs in a spiralling path to shine in the eyes. *Shen* is the least material of the treasures and is the celestial spark that ignites the functioning of the other two.

In relating the three treasures, *jing* is more on the physical solid plane, *shen* is the consciousness that is identified with the mind and the senses and the least tangible of the three, while *qi* is the underlying intermediate substance that links the other two. *Jing*, *qi* and *shen* are fundamentally the same entities inhabiting different forms. The mutability of water serves as an analogy with its liquid phase corresponding to *qi*, vapour to *shen* and denser ice to *jing*. In order to grasp *qi gong* breathing, it is important to approach this concept of the interchangeability of the treasures, for the constructs of Taoism are based on transformation of the three substances into each other. In this process, breath is a direct manifestation of the *qi* that is converted into *jing* and *shen* via the respiratory, corporeal and mental coordination of *qi gong*.

QI CULTIVATION AND THE THREE DAN TIANS

How does one cultivate *qi*? In *qi gong*, the mind, governed by the spirit, is conveyed through visualization and breath to the locality known as the lower *dan tian*. This is the gathering and storage point of *qi*. One of the goals of *qi gong* breathing is to conduct *jing* from the kidneys to the lower *dan tian* where it is converted to *qi* for health, vitality, or spiritual evolution. This conversion of *jing* to *qi* is brought about in the lower *dan tian* through further catalytic action of the breath. The lower *dan tian* is considered the centre of gravity and the physical focal point of the body. It is called the 'elixir field' and is situated midway between the navel and the pubic bone. Some *qi gong* texts note its anatomical centre at two finger widths below the navel, level with the acupuncture point, *Ren 6* (see Figure 10.1). Other texts locate it four finger widths below the navel at *Ren 4*. The *dan tian* is deep from the surface of the body, but closer to the belly than the back.

There are two other *dan tians* that serve as destinations for the path of *qi* in the anatomical landscape. The middle *dan tian* is located in the centre of the chest on the sternum. The point association is *Ren* 17. However, in *qi gong* practice, when moving the breath, the middle *dan tian* is often associated with the upper abdomen and the solar plexus. The corresponding point, *Ren* 12, is located a hand width above the navel. The third *dan tian* (*yintang*), is located between the eyebrows. It is also called the third eye and is especially affiliated with the *shen*.

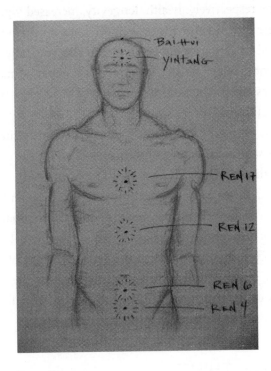

Figure 10.1

In the practice of *qi gong*, *qi* is conducted through an intricate network called meridians. There are 12 major meridians that connect to the major organ systems of the body and eight extra meridians, which function as reservoirs for *qi*. The meridians are analogous to waterways with the fluid like *qi* transporting vitality to the entire body. These meridians also guide blood to moisten and nourish the body. *Qi* and blood rise to the surface of the skin at points where the interior can be affected through acupuncture needles or finger pressure. Since *qi* is transmutable to *shen*, the meridian system forms a geometric network in the body where life force and spirit potentially converge.

CATEGORIES OF QI GONG

The kind of *qi gong* engaged in and the goal sought determine the desired *qi* flow patterns and breathing techniques required; this in turn determines how the three treasures are cultivated and transmuted. The principle categories of *qi gong* include medical – with forms that vary according to the kind of illness encountered – and martial arts – with hard forms such as kung fu and soft forms like tai chi. There is also spiritual *qi gong*, often with a decidedly Buddhist underpinning. The primary aims of *qi gong* are, respectively: health, longevity, increased vigour and spiritual enlightenment. These categories of *qi gong* are horizontally complex in their plurality of styles as developed in various schools. *Qi gong* is also vertically dense in the several disciplines that come under its rubric such as a number of martial arts, massage, stretching exercises and meditation. All varieties of *qi gong* can be classified as either external or internal forms.

External forms of *qi gong* include such practices as stretching, martial arts, acupuncture and massage that focuses on utilizing *qi* to fortify the physical body. In these methods *qi* that is stimulated on the surface of the body moves to the interior. By contrast, internal forms work to directly strengthen the *qi* in the body centres and organs. Internal forms include various methods of breathing that are used to nourish and circulate the *qi* through the meridians, organs, the physical body and the *shen* or spiritual body. In cyclical fashion, due to the Taoist principle of balance, both forms benefit each other synergistically when practised sequentially. In that progression, internal *qi gong* is considered more advanced since it potentially moves beyond the physical body into spiritual realms.

MODES OF BREATHING

There are two primary kinds of breathing that concern internal *qi gong*: abdominal and reverse.

In abdominal breathing the relaxed belly moves out during inhalation and in during exhalation. Abdominal breathing recovers how a baby breathes. The direction here is to maintain a Buddha belly. Both the area above and below the navel remains open to the movement of breath: the upper abdomen corresponding to the solar plexus and the lower *dan tian* parallelling the region below the navel where *qi* is refined and stored.

Reverse breathing is the opposite of abdominal breathing. In this case, the abdominal area moves inward on the incoming breath and moves outward on the outgoing breath. Moving the abdomen in lifts the diaphragm on the inhalation so that contact is made with the *Chong* meridian. This meridian is the main reservoir for *qi*.

In Taoist anatomy, it runs through the spine. Energetically it is viewed as penetrating and connecting all three *dan tians*. In reverse breathing, during inhalation, the *Chong* is stimulated to move *qi* from the lower to the higher dan tians. Then, after the *qi* rises to its peak, this flow of energy reverses, travelling downward from the upper to the lower *dan tian* on the outgoing breath. During this exhalation, the belly expands in order to spread the *qi* through the lower *dan tian* so as to recharge it. With reverse breathing, *qi gong* masters advise the application of mindful action in order to avoid excessive tension. Thus, economy of effort is valued regarding organization of breath and muscular contractions.

It should be noted that reversed breathing is a specialized kind of respiration that is used to build and increase *qi* concentration and flow. This kind of breathing relates to the kind of exertion necessary for lifting a heavy object with the exception that the energy is not discharged but stored and spread through the centre. It corresponds to a heightened state of energy where one doesn't collapse on exhalation and even gains a sense of expansion. While there may be considerable distinctions in technique, reverse breathing compares with the kind of stamina and breath lengthening approaches taught in the western setting for the extraordinary demands of heightened theatrical speaking and singing. This comparison is only on principle since western training for actors and singers, even when utilizing such methods as rib reserve, adheres to an abdominal breathing blueprint. For *qi gong* practitioners as well, it is important to acknowledge that relaxed abdominal breathing is the default system relied on during everyday restful and active states.

Most *qi gong* instruction involves nasal breathing, sometimes with an active thought of drawing the *qi* down to the bottom of the belly. In some kinds of *qi gong* where clearing pathological excess is the goal, expelling toxins through the mouth occurs. For the more meditative sequences in *qi gong* where the focus is on the lower *dan tian* the breathing is through the nose.

Each organ system has its own *qi* direction and in the case of the Lung, which governs respiration, the movement is down. Pathological lung conditions, such as asthma, involve the rebellious upward flow of *qi* causing congestion in the chest. That is why in *qi gong* practice, one is instructed to breathe down to the bottom of the feet. One master, C.K. Chu, describes the breath as 'long, deep, small, smooth' (Eternal 14). The breath is lengthened to match the slower cycles of nature's rhythm. The ancient Taoists believed this alignment of breath rate with nature would lead to slower physical deterioration and greater longevity. Slowing down the breath and making it deeper improves oxygenation of the blood, restoring the cells and nourishing the *qi*. The rationale behind keeping the breath small configures with economy of effort and offsets the tendency of heavy breathing, which the Taoist thought would over tax the lungs. Finally, the concept of smoothness requires a fluid breath without choppiness. Altering the breath's rate, depth, quantity and quality transforms the body's *qi*, *jing* and *shen* to affect emotions, as well as, mental and spiritual states.

LINKING QI GONG AND VOICE

In combining *qi gong* theory with western voice practice one must acknowledge discrepancies. Breath holding, for example, is one technique practised in some kinds of *qi gong* that western voice teachers usually discourage. Rather than straining to contain the wide complexity of *qi gong* technology within the scope of a voice warm-up, it is more profitable to regard specific types of *qi gong* that converse more freely with western breathing practices resulting in a natural, unforced affinity. Due to the common ground shared with touch, there is a potential synergy between voice work and the branch of *qi gong* concerned with massage. This is particularly true of self-massage where some of the techniques can be incorporated into a personal tune-up without the need for a professional body worker or partner.

The combination proposed is not so unorthodox if one considers the historical precedent evident in the adaptations *qi gong* underwent due to the imports of Hindu and Buddhist systems from India. Additionally, since then, *qi gong*, like a living language, though ancient, has spawned many metamorphoses as new innovations and styles grow from the creative variations of Taoist and Buddhist schools. This provides some basis for experimentation when guided by a reverence for the tradition. One *qi gong* master, Dr Yang Jwing-Ming, offers an invitation when he writes, 'Different cultures from different races finally have a chance to look at each other. It is time for us to open our minds to other cultures and even adopt their good parts' (1991, p. 13). While honouring the Immortals of the past, Taoists firmly live in the present and acknowledge the need for mastery of contemporary skills, if only to ultimately abandon them for a more spiritual path. But it should also be noted that *qi gong* massage has roots in empiricism as a therapeutic method that preceded imported spiritual influences.

Qi gong self massage is an external form, since the application is from the exterior to the interior. Through a variety of techniques involving tactility, *qi* is raised up on the superficial layers of the body and transported to the internal viscera. Through breath the mind fine-tunes to the sensations engendered to create a communicative network that balances and enlivens the whole organism. Since *qi gong* massage is a method of self-diagnosis, this purpose can extend to a practitioner when reading and navigating the body in order to discharge stressful holding patterns on dermal, muscular and visceral levels. If you enliven the *qi*, there is also a potential for enlivening the *shen* due to their transmutability. Since healthy *qi* flows rather than stagnates and such fluidity activates and clears the mind, one becomes more sensitized to the messages of the body. This allows the area touched to dictate the kind of approach required. Ideally, animation of mind or *shen* increases self-awareness in an open, sensuous circuitry rather than in the closed way that characterizes self-consciousness.

In traditional Chinese medicine, the Lung governs the skin, respiration and the vigour of the voice. While *qi gong* massage is often done without a vocal component, the partnering of touch and deep breathing with sound may further texture the experience with a potentiating effect. When releasing sound, root it in the lower *dan tian*, visualize and sense the currents of vibration, clarify the arrival points on the body. Later, experiment with vibrations radiating off the points like transmitting stations to specific places around the room, or a partner. The sound can follow a familiar voice approach or can be more improvisational. In the latter case, once familiar with the massage, think of keeping the sound going using vowels, hums and occasionally consonants in order to create a jam session of vibration and body awareness. Let the fingers and skin communicate through the sound, each one imparting energy to the other.

What follows is an introduction to a detailed, experimental self-massage of the whole body. One of the advantages of self-massage over acupuncture and partnered bodywork is that self-massage can be done practically anywhere. With the inclusion of voice, these exercises are best done in a quiet, private environment and they can serve as a warm-up before a speaking engagement. Traditionally, *qi gong* is done in the morning to start the day. But self-massage can be adapted to circumstances as necessary. Because self-massage is often done for a therapeutic effect, timing may be based on achieving the desired outcome of healing. Repeat each exercise until a warm glowing sensation is achieved in the area massaged. Generally, stop massaging if the arms or hands are getting fatigued. As more familiarity is built, it is best to improvize with the time spent on each exercise, as one begins to listen to the promptings of the body and the mind. In adapting *qi gong* self-massage to sound, it is preferable to let the breath effortlessly enter through the mouth rather than the nose particularly for communication, when receiving and sending energy to a partner. Please note that the benefits listed for these exercises are drawn from traditional Taoism and are not intended to substitute for medical advice.

QI GONG SELF-MASSAGE WITH SOUND: HEAD
Opening

Title:	Invigorating the hands
Aim:	To warm the hands by bringing *qi* and intention into them.
How:	• Rub the palms together vigorously while intermittently pausing to blow the body's heated outgoing breath on them.

Title:	Sensing the *Qi* Ball
Aim:	Connect the mind with the qi flow between the hands.
How:	• Close your eyes.

• Spread your hands slightly apart.

• Keep your palms facing each other while bringing them together until they touch.

• Gradually move the hands apart with the palms facing each other and keep the feeling of the energy between them.

• Imagine a ball of energy or light balanced between the two hands.

• Spend a minimum of one or two minutes sensing the *qi* ball. The ball, however, can be held for several minutes.

Head

Title:	Stimulating the scalp
Aim:	Next, use a rubbing technique with circular motion. The purpose of rubbing is to soothe the muscles, enhance *qi* and blood circulation and to dissipate stagnant *qi* so that the body can remove it.
How:	• Vigorously use the fingertips to massage the scalp.

• Avoid scratching with the fingernails. Use the tips to deeply rub.

• Continue for 15 to 30 seconds.

Title:	Rubbing the heavenly gate
Aim:	Massaging this point can alleviate headache and improve the nervous system.
How:	• Locate *Du* 20 (*baihui*). The point is at the top of the head, at the intersection of two imaginary lines: one drawn up from the apexes of the ears and the other line between the tip of the nose and the base of the skull. The point is named for the one hundred meridians that converge at this site.

How:
- Bring your dominant hand up to the crown and gently but firmly massage the area.
- Rub in a circular manner.
- While rubbing send several hums to your lips and feel the vibrations at the crown of your head.
- Repeat a minimum of three rotations, building up to 12 or more circles.

Title: Tapping the head

Aim: Knocking the head lightly can help to sharpen the thinking.

How:
- With fists gently tap the head to clear the mind and stimulate the scalp.
- Add hums to this circular tapping.
- Explore opening and closing the lips; closed lips build internal energy and opening them releases the energized sound and with it, tensions.
- Repeat a minimum of three times.

Title: Massaging the temples

Aim: To reduce stress and soothe the nerves

How:
- Massage the hollow of the temples (*taiyang*) with knuckles of index fingers centrifugally moving the circles backward to release pressure from the inside for dispersal to the outside.
- Circle until the area feels soothed and stress-free.

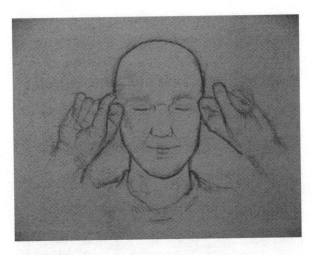

Figure 10.2

Eyes

Title: Opening the windows of the *shen*

Aim: To clear the vision, soften the eyes and brighten the spirit.

How:
- Press all the points around the eye orbits with fingertips or thumbs being careful not to poke the eye.

- Rub both hands together until they are warm.

- Then cover your closed eyes with the palms. Repeat this a few times to send healing *qi* into the eye area.

- Add open vowel sounds or hums.

How:
- Start with the palms covering the closed eyes. Send *qi* into your eyes from your hands and send sound vibrations into the eyes on a hum from the lower *dan tian*.

- While slowly opening the eyes gradually move the palms away out in front of the eyes. Move the hands out as far as you can while keeping contact with the *qi* flowing into the eyes and the vibrations streaming gently out from the eyes.

Nose

Title: Opening the nose

Aim: There are three meridians running through the nose: the *Du*, the master meridian for the yang of the entire body, the stomach and the large intestine. Rubbing the nose moves the organ *qi* of these associated meridians. It also opens the sinuses. Additionally, the lung governs the nose; therefore, a strong nose benefits the voice.

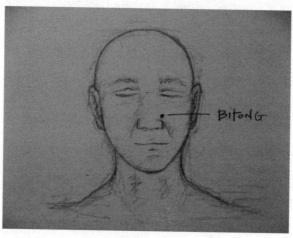

Figure 10.3

How:
- Give gentle fingertip acupressure alongside the nose to *bitong*, releasing sound spontaneously.
- With the backs of the thumbs vigorously massage up and down the area just lateral to the sides of the nose, adding hums. Here, explore letting the air in through the nose to clear the passageways for the sound that will follow.
- Repeat several times until the breath flows easily through the nose and the skin gets warm.

Mouth

Title: Circling the lips

Aim: Since the meridians most involved with digestion, the stomach and the spleen, connect to the mouth, this exercise is utilized to improve that function.

How:
- Purse lips into a pucker and move in a circle. Then open the lips.
- Repeat on a hum.
- Repeat circle in other direction. Then open the lips.
- Repeat on a hum in this direction.
- Repeat a minimum of three times in each direction.

Title: Pressing the gums

Aim: This exercise stimulates the most yin and most yang channels accessed through *Ren* 24 and *Du* 26. It is also considered a stimulant to digestion and, therefore, can be done after meals.

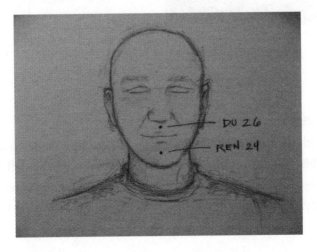

Figure 10.4

How: • Use fingertips to drum around upper and lower gums. Add hums or spontaneous vowel sounds.

• Change the direction of the drumming.

• Repeat a minimum of three times in each direction.

Jaw

Title: Softening the jaw

Aim: Here the purpose is to dissipate accumulated jaw stress.

How: • Give acupressure to Stomach 6, the bulge muscle of the jaw, called the masseter.

• Use fingertips with small circular motions on Small Intestine 19. These are two bilateral points just between the tragus and the mandibular joint. Send vibrations via several hums to soften the jaw. Keep the teeth unclenched when doing this exercise.

• Repeat several times until the area feels soft, open and relaxed.

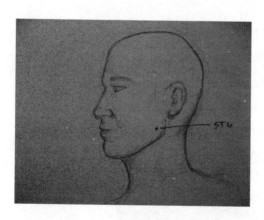

Figure 10.5

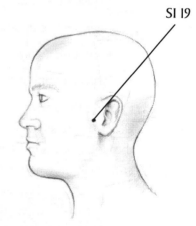

Figure 10.6

Ears

Title: Pounding the celestial drum

Aim: To both tone and relax the inner ear. Because the kidney governs the ear, this exercise is utilized to strengthen that organ as well as the hearing. Additionally, the ear is considered the human antenna to infinity. Ideally, permit receptivity in the silence following the exercise.

How:
- Cover both ears with each hand (fingers facing back towards each other).

- Flick fingers rapidly on occipital bone.

- Then suddenly bring palms off of ears to sharpen your hearing.

- Repeat the process with sound, visualizing the vibrations coming up from the lower *dan tian* and filling the head. While beating the celestial drum, start on a hum then explore opening the lips keeping your contact with the lower *dan tian* and letting that energy spread to the middle and upper *dan tians*.

- Open your lips, keeping the sound going as you release your hands from your ears.

- Repeat a minimum of three times.

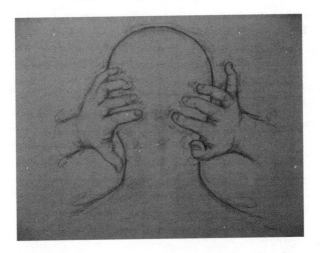

Figure 10.7

In *qi gong* self-massage with sound, it is the mind, the manifestation of spirit, that is important in its ability to direct the flow of *qi* and vibrations through visualization, to sense the interior and periphery of the body, to make creative choices based on an orchestration of sensory, imagistic and visceral energies. These vibrations become inseparable from the gut instincts as well as the breath that both embodies them and gives them flight.

BIBLIOGRAPHY

Chang, Stephen (1986) *The Complete System of Self-Healing: Internal Exercises.* San Francisco: Tao.

Cheng, Xinnong (ed.) (1987) *Chinese Acupuncture and Moxibustion.* Beijing: Foreign Language Press.

Chia, Mantak (1986) *Iron Shirt Chi Kung I.* Huntington, New York: Healing Tao.

Chia, Mantak (1986) *Chi Self-Massage.* Huntington, New York: Healing Tao.

Chu, C.K. (2003) *Eternal Spring Chi Kung.* Forest Hills Station, NY: Sunflower.

Chu, C.K. (2002) *Chu Meditation: A Step by Step Guide.* Forest Hills Station, NY: Sunflower.

de Langre, Jacques (1974) *The First Book of Do/-In.* Hollywood: Happiness Press.

de Langre, Jacques (1976) *The Second Book of Do/-In.* Magalia, CA: Happiness Press.

Deng, Ming-Dao (1990) *Scholar Warrior: An Introduction to the Tao in Everyday life.* New York: HarperCollins.

Deng, Ming-Dao (1983) *The Wandering Taoist.* New York: HarperCollins.

Hon, Sat Chuen (2003) *Taoist Qigong for Health and Vitality.* Boston: Shambhala.

Kaptchuk, Ted J. (1983) *The Web That Has No Weaver: Understanding Chinese Medicine.* New York: Congdon & Weed.

Kushi, Michio (1979) *The Book of Do/-In: Exercise for Physical and Spiritual Development.* Tokyo: Japan Publications.

Lade, Arnie (1989) *Acupuncture Points: Images and Functions.* Seattle: Eastland Press.

Maciocia, Giovanni (1989) *The Foundation of Chinese Medicine: A Comprehensive Text for Acupuncturists and Herbalists.* Edinburgh: Churchill Livingstone.

Sioux, Lily (1975) *Chi Kung: The Mastering of the Unseen Life Force.* Rutland, Vermont: Charles E. Tuttle.

Yang, Jwing-Ming (1991) *Muscle/Tendon Changing and Marrow/Brain Washing Chi Kung: The Secret of Youth.* Jamaica Plain, MA: YMAA.

Zhang, Yu Huan and Ken Rose (2001) *A Brief History of Qi.* Brookline, MA: Paradigm.

CHAPTER 11

Integrated Movement Practices and the Breath

DEBBIE GREEN

In this chapter, I use the template of my first and second year BA Acting Pathway movement curriculum, a developmental structure, to offer the experience of holistic practice and well-being to seekers of the authentic self through movement and breath. The word 'actor' will appear throughout the chapter as it is through working with actors that the depth of the work has been revealed and it has been that throughout history, theatre has revealed ourselves to ourselves...

I step forward and join my feet, sweeping my hands passed my upper chest and turn the palms down, turn my feet out, sink into a plié, curve forward to touch the floor and then my forehead with my hands, bring my hands to my solar plexus/heart and as I rise once more I open my arms forward and then outward, join the hands again in prayer position opposite my left breast and sink into my left hip, my turned out left leg and foot. I am sinking into the 'Tribhanga Paada' (three-bend) of Odissi, the North Eastern Indian classical dance form.

And this was inspiration. This was 'coming home' into my body and more particularly into my female body after years of western dance. It was about my movement being allowed to follow the curves of my female form, about giving into my waist, sinking into my female hips, about my feet settling into the earth and it was about yielding to my weight and breath. My classical ballet trained body 'got' the 'style', but I understand now how long it had taken me as a professional dancer to find my weight, my base and breath. And slowly I began to understand and deconstruct my classical ballet training, which I had allowed to inhibit my inner sense of dance. The outside was so much stronger than the inside. The namaska of Odissi follows breath; when you rest in the final Tribhanga you have breathed; the movements follow the breath. The movement sequence has the ease of a natural form. I also knew the Chouka Paada, the square position, or as it was taught to me, the male position. I came to know these as the lasya (delicate) as opposed to the tandava (vigorous) and I had discovered oppositions. I had gained an analytical awareness of the two polarities and therefore the range in between and since have gone on exploring 'energy'; male and female principles perhaps, hard and soft energy; yin and yang; Barba's 'Animus and Anima – the temperatures of the energy' (Barba 1991, p. 61).

And I came to a point when I did not know what to do with this Indian dance form – the prospect of continuing the cycle of study and performance seemed purposeless unless I embraced the dance culture entirely into my life. So, I left the dances behind, but knew that I had the dance in my being. I had found my feet and begun to find teaching work and I found teaching actors.

The sensual experience changed me. And it went on working. I found more work that rooted me and that gave me time and breath.

I found myself returned to my body or perhaps given my body through the classical Indian dance. This was my way in and one that I had not asked to find except by choosing the dynamic and sensual dance form that I had. By doing this unconsciously (I fell in love with what I saw on the stage), I had offered myself the potential for this homecoming. I had bound myself for years with the high and shallow breathing of an unaware trained classical ballet dancer, not understanding the natural way of my breath and its connection with the movement and therefore its potential expressivity. This sense of awareness, of presence and thus of working with breath, yield and give, needed channelling into my movement work for the actor.

The sensual experience of movement for actors is one that I offer to first and second year acting students. The fundamental work is based on the integration of breath and movement. There is a balance to be found between learning and practising form and the application of the experience into free form, whilst guiding the students to relinquish inhibition and uncertainty, always encouraging them to breathe the form so that it can move them. The gesture/movement here happens on the out-breath; followed by rest on the in-breath. Through any movement variation in this sequence, connection to personal breath is key.

A potent variation, with students lying on the floor for the duration, can provide a seminal moment when they speak of the sensuality experienced through the work, when they discover that their movement is both liquid and muscular and that each quality is powerful and necessary in and of itself. The experience of sensuality is equally important to all students regardless of previous movement training. So often the joints, particularly at the ankle, are rigid which means that the legs up to the hips are tight. The sensual body is beautiful and we are affected by both sensuality and beauty. To access the subtle use of different qualities, rhythms and emotions, habitual tension habits must be released and can be released through this work. Not all students achieve the same level of sensuality but each can enhance their own movement facility through understanding its strength when measured against this other quality.

Slowly, through the developing self-awareness, the student learns about the place of neutrality, this place of potential, of alertness, of physical attention and, primarily in the training, of postural alignment. The aim is to find the state of 'being', which is one of total 'availability'. This requires internal relaxation via precise re-alignment of the body, giving an entirely free diaphragm, but also freedom of physical expression into the space around the body. Breath begins to move in and out of the body more freely.

My Movement Fundamental work develops awareness of the subtle, sensual messages received through conscious mobilizing of the body through breath. Slowly the student finds and releases blocks to the flow of energy through the body and begins to work with an integrated sense of the body – lower half to upper half. The work demands the discipline of inner attention and 'listening in' to the body and allowing the body weight to open up areas of physicality denied when the upper half is carrying too much energy and effort. The released voice results incidentally or accidentally, from this physical discovery in the movement classes.

I teach holistically not allowing the head supremacy over the body but bringing the head and body relationship back into balance. We behave and see the world with such control if we hold the neck and head. Our responses and action are not embodied. How can we get the 'mind into the body and out of the head'? Dr Candace Pert, pharmacologist of international repute and best known for her research into how the body-mind functions as a single psychosomatic network of information molecules that control health and physiology, describes how 'your brain is actually a "mobile brain" that moves throughout your entire body – since it is located in all places at once and not just in the head' (Pert 1997, pp. 9-10)!

As the students watch each other in the Contact Improvisation classes (a duo-dance improvisation through physical contact/touch, which creates a frame for observing the functions of the body's reflexes), it is so easy to see when those who are working in the space are planning the next move, not heeding the touch which is happening in the moment. And so, we go back to base and try to leave this tentative and ponderous over-sensing behind – or bust through it and reveal it experientially.

What informs my particular approach to movement teaching is the power 'in' the body – the alive and awake presence; that can possess a powerful stride, an animal quality, beauty of the spine in alignment and an inner connection to stillness (which has fullness); it can connect to the ground and to breath through release; that is, being in the body in the moment. Through my movement work with acting students, I respond eagerly to Pert's understanding that, 'Your body-mind intelligently guides what you perceive as "life itself"' (Pert 1997, pp. 9–10)!

The student learns to recognize the need to be in the 'present', or in the now, or in the moment. David Abram in his book *The Spell of the Sensuous* draws on an eclectic mix of sources – the philosophy of Merleau-Ponty, Balinese shamanism, Apache storytelling and his own experience as an accomplished magician – as he defines this 'present' as a greater thing than just a tense, explaining that 'the present has determined itself as presence only by taking on the precise contours of the visible landscape that enfold us. We are now free to look around us, in this vast terrain, for the place of the past and of the future' (Abram 1997, p. 209).

Implicit for performance then is the notion of stillness, power, quiet and clarity which is at the core of presence. Thus our performing body, responding to stimuli from moment to moment, allows us to empty through the out-breath and with the ebb and flow of energy and breath, the student learns about the state of empty fullness.

Into the variations of movement and breath explorations, we add the Bartenieff Fundamentals through which I encourage the quality of ease and flow, the release of held muscles and joints, the contrast of softness and strength and the power of liquidity. There is a sense of space created through the work and a growing connection to the floor. This experiential knowledge is taken into the feet when upright, so that the developing malleability and sensitivity, as well as, the tone of the extremities, come into relationship with the floor.

Part of that first term's work is to find centre and experience moving from this, understanding the impulse from gathering into the centre to move outwards from the centre (scattering) from a rooted, down to earth place and an engaged body that is always ready for action. As I watch the students' progress through the sequence, I am reminded of the Qigong practitioner moving very slowly, almost imperceptibly and then so fast, all his movement focused within his kinesphere (personal space around the body to the limit of reach of extremities) while the liquidity of the movement manifests itself in the flow of energy. In students, soft flow can so easily be misinterpreted as collapse, weakness and non-tone of the muscles. This energy is ours to manipulate through the performance; it is there to be tapped – a ceaseless flow – to be shaped. In contrast, full energy can be misinterpreted as push, over exertion that traps and inhibits the movement which then remains bound and stuck.

We explore soft martial arts, Yoga and Pilates (method of body conditioning which includes stretching and strengthening exercises); slow exercises that allow time to focus on and open up specific areas of the body. Students are encouraged to

> feel the in-breath in the back – opening the shoulder blades and ribs out from the spine like angel wings; like eagle wings. Feel the expansion of the ribs at the back through the in-breath and the width and openness in the back.

I invite the students to move and speak from this sensual experience of the upper back. The lower back can be opened and stretched through, for instance, the Pilates spine stretch, rolling like a ball, the cat curl of both Yoga and Pilates, through Bartenieff Fundamentals, culminating in the movement improvisation I introduce from the contact between the hand of one partner and the sacrum of the other.

The expiratory breath can be explored through Pilates. Total forced expiratory actions are assisted by the Rectus Abdominis and the student can easily feel and access this muscle, working deep in the pelvic region pressing towards the spine. The Transversus Abdominis is a main player here in the core strength work too, but full abdominal muscle co-contraction is really how it feels to the students. Pilates develops core strength and stabilizes the hips. The sensation of the 'pulling up of the abdominal muscles deep into the body under the ribs' and 'softening the lower front ribs gently down to the waist' as well as softening the chest is powerful. The pelvic tilt using the 'abdominal scoop' is also crucial in protecting the spine. This is balanced with the imagery of the work of the Iliopsoas – the postural muscles of the lower back and pelvis – which can offer a less aggressive approach to the support used by the actor. The wonder of balance, inner lift and poise and the muscular strength on a rise on the balls of the feet can be experienced when these muscles and the pelvic tilt are consciously recruited. It is essential that the student knows both the release of the abdominal muscles as well as the support that is gained through abdominal strength. Following a Pilates and Yoga based warm-up students frequently comment on how amazing their postures and voices are, how connected to the breath they feel.

There is ongoing exploration and a gradual heightening of the sensation of being upright with the need to feel both uprightness and downwardness; the 'feel' of the vertical within ourselves. Images that come to mind are of gothic church architecture with its awe inspiring height and verticality, or of trees and their rooted stillness. Either of these can trigger movement within that begins to connect us to our height/

length and to the breath of the vertical, the breath and sensation of the abstract infinite line up and down through the spine.

It is the power 'in' the body, as well as, 'of' the body, that all acting students need to explore and we can, even momentarily sense the completeness and openness truly of ourselves. We want to be able to take our life/primal/creative force, or our vitality, on to the stage, knowing that we can accentuate one or the other energy, i.e. Animus and Anima and allowing this to move throughout an open body, a released pelvis and a backbone. This life energy can be seen as 'presence', as energy coursing through the three dimensionality of the performer who uses/plays this efficiently and effectively, so that the body is alive for the audience. Barba describes presence, or performer's energy, as a combination of 'nervous and muscular power' (Barba 1991, p. 74). The performer allows this much energy out for this moment and contains it here and releases it explosively there and crucial to this control are intention, breath and release.

When the work hits home, there is a sense that you are sitting inside the work by allowing yourself to get out of the way, neither collapsing nor pushing the effect, but 'sinking the mind', letting go to the task and finding the intention from the centre of the weight. 'Where the foot goes there the belly goes; you do not leave yourself behind.'

There is always a need to return to the feet. I learned to really consider mine through finding my 'Odissi feet' that needed to be both accurately percussive and dextrous, working on stone floors and so needed to remain released. Sue Weston, T'ai-Chi teacher and initiator of Relaxing The Mind, provided me with further insights through practice of the 'metal detector over the ground' quality of the feet and their placing on the ground from the heel to the toes in the T'ai-Chi slow walk. Most importantly I came to understand the feet through the wonderful images of the 'bubbling well point' in the middle of the sole of the foot and the triangle made by the points under the big and little toe joints and the middle of the heel. I once watched a camel's feet softly spread out in the sand in the desert of Rajasthan as the weight was transferred into it. Like this vivid image, I truly felt my own feet once I stepped out of pointe shoes, allowing them to spread on the floor and really take my weight.

How complicated it seems at first, even at the end of the first year of training, to maintain grounding in the even and rhythmic beat of the feet loping in the ground combined with the flow of the torso in the first of Gabrielle Roth's five rhythms – 'Flowing'. The pulse that the feet must continually maintain keeps the movement rooted with the weight dropped into the feet.

Finding and developing 'the sensual and energetic body' takes time and the student has to understand that it is a drip feed learning process as opposed to fast track learning based on result. It demands inner attention, time to allow things to happen and a relish for detail. It demands commitment, discipline, professionalism and generosity of self. It demands sophistication, personal self-awareness, curiosity about one's body, about the fundamental movement of the acting body and a hunger to engage with the experiential process that these demand. Said a student about his movement studies:

> Funny how of all the things I did at Central, instead of acting…all your Tai-chi, Bartenieff and Contact Improvisation work have been endlessly enriching for me in my development as a performer…I always felt that work we did with you in that room in the Winch was making a subtle but profound difference to me at a level I couldn't quite understand. Now I realise that it was my body re-establishing a more balanced relationship with my overbearing mind! (Harders, Email, 19 April 2005)

Judgmental and censoring mentality from inhibiting social and personal mores can be shifted into an absorbed and open attitude. Students have to want to find out about every moment of their inhalation and exhalation. They learn to see what it 'gives off' in others and therefore what this offers them as well. Working on the development of a physical sensuality cannot survive an inattentive or impatient approach, preconceived ideas of and associations to the movement or, indeed, a prescriptive notion of movement. Movement is a delicate business because its site is the body. When there is real engagement with the work, there is beauty because the students are open and innocent, working in an uncomplicated way towards embodiment, making an investment in detail as they bring themselves utterly to the work.

I came home into my female body through a dance form that is earth based as opposed to the air based classical ballet I had grown up with. I embraced this dance form that encompasses both male and female characters, albeit deities and demands that the dancer takes on both male and female stylized characters. Reflecting upon my Odissi dance, upon energy and how I softened muscular control, I became aware of the developing relationship I had in my own body with different 'temperatures' of energy. This awareness gave me access into structuring a Movement Fundamental curriculum in which I emphasize a soft yielding quality as counterbalance to a hard, muscular quality. Of course, both ends of the spectrum of hard and soft are needed by both sexes. Each gender can struggle with both, but in my class, 'masculine' and 'feminine' are understood as simply qualities to be explored. The energetic and sensual body means that the body can be as large and as heavy, or as small and light, as it actually is and can take the whole of the space that it actually needs and more and less, but with sensitivity and by being awake to itself, the outside informed by the inside through the breath.

EXERCISES

Title: 'Smelling the rose': suspension and fall

Aim: To experience yielding to the dynamic of weight through breath. It is important that you are warmed up prior to doing this exercise and do it up to six times each to start with, adding to it in gentle stages, so that the integrity and quality of the work are the priority. It is worth starting this work on large mats with space around each couple, but eventually this exercise can be achieved on the wooden, studio floor.

Step I: Suspension and fall

• Stand opposite and facing your partner. Maintain a rooted and wide stance.

• Each using one arm, grasp opposite wrists.

• Each take your weight back, holding wrists, so that you are pulling away from each other. Make certain that the back is rounded – producing that 'C' curve of the spine – as you do so.

• Use the impetus of the pulling away from each other to bring yourself upright once again.

• Release the wrist grasp and let the arm travel upwards above your head with the inhalation, as if trying to wring/stretch out the very last drop of scent that can be inhaled from a perfumed rose.

• On the exhalation, the other arm reaches downward and then up to reach for the partner's other wrist, as response to suspension of the inhalation.

• Still on the exhale, fall so that you allow the body weight to drop back using the grasp of the partner's wrist to catch this. Be certain to have some physical yield, give and elasticity, rather than collapse or tense muscular hold. This ensures that the actual work is a suspension and fall, resulting in the lightness that is the hallmark of this exercise when observed. This can, of course, be tiring to do for any length of time and yet it looks so easy.

Step 2: On the floor

The 'Suspension and Fall' can be developed so that you allow your partner to sink into the floor.

- Still facing your partner, using one arm, grab opposite wrists.

- With the pull of weight, one of you controls the other's descent through the grasp of the wrist, to sitting and then lying.

- As you walk towards, to the side and then past your partner on the floor, release her/his hand to walk around behind her/him. Make sure that the movement is a response to this momentum and the breath while you walk around your partner.

- On the exhale, grasp your partner's other wrist and hand.

- On the inhale, pull your partner up.

- Suspend or hold this pose, but not the breath.

- Now let the other partner descend to the floor by following steps one through six.

- Repeat these steps to create a seesaw action.

Title: Shifting three-bend exercise: suitable for a non-actor. *The experience of the following exercise is reminiscent of the Tribhanga Paada of the classical Indian dance form, Odissi – the three bend posture of lasya, or delicate or feminine – but it is adapted from a Qigong exercise whose similarity struck me:*

Aim: To experience yielding to the dynamic of weight through the breath. The exercise simply continues; repetition as a key to learning through the movement itself. This can be done in any working space and is most satisfying when working as a group.

- Stand with legs and feet parallel and under your hips, facing front, with the 'intention' in the belly directed to the front where it remains focused throughout the exercise. With the hip bones and belly remaining facing to the front all the time during the exercise, the pelvis simply swings/shifts from side to side allowing your sacrum and tail bone to drop straight down to the floor. If you were lying on the floor you could experience the lateral shift of the hips/pelvis, really imagining that they can move to the side in a straight line so that there is not a distortion in the hips. Otherwise, if you allow the hip to turn away from the front in the exercise, the work has a completely different meaning and quality, losing the openness and power of working from centre.

- Breathe in to prepare.

- Breathe out and sink down into your left leg and foot, bending the knee, keeping the toes loosely in line with the heel at about 12 o'clock, allowing the left hip to shift to the side, keeping the hip bones facing the front and in response turning out the right leg in the hip, knee facing to the right and resting the ball of the foot on the ground. Your torso responds to this shift of the hip and the sinking into it, by gathering at the waist, i.e. a concertinaing of the waist; you allow the waist to move in response to the breath, with the lower side rib softly squeezing towards the hip on the same side. The spine is malleable and the head, as part of your spine, physically responds to this movement with a slight shift also from side to side of the chin, in relation to the shift of the hip on the same side.

- Breathe in and feel the rising inside as you pass through the starting position of the torso and legs.

- Breathe out and slip into the right hip and leg, bending the knee and keeping the hip bones facing front, with the foot loosely pivoting/swivelling on the ball to enable this and then landing on the whole foot with the heel down, the foot at about 12 o'clock, as it becomes the supporting foot, turning out the left leg in the hip, knee facing to the left and resting the ball of the left foot on the ground.

- This exercise continues on alternate sides, following the gentle rise and fall of breath, with your body yielding to this rhythm, your arms simply hanging down to your sides. The hip slides to the side on the out-breath and the rise through 'neutral' occurs on the in-breath, in order that on the next breath out, you can slip into the hip on the other side. Each of the movements integrates with the breath through the rise and fall of the transfer of weight from one foot to the other as the feet swivel, either as support with the toes in front of the heel at 12 o'clock or, with the knee turned out to the side in response to the foot pivoting on the ball and the heel lifting from the floor. The movement of your feet can be likened to the action of 'massaging the feet in the ground', or 'kneading dough' or 'treading grapes'.

- The exercise simply continues; repetition as a key to learning through the movement itself.

Title: The Jellyfish from Wilhelm Reich
Aim: Deep breathing and opening of the lower body.

This can be repeated for up to five minutes and then longer as the body accustoms itself to the experience and moves through any muscular shaking of the legs that may occur. This exercise needs a mat and a support to the back of the head if there is a habit of raising the chin when lying.

- Lie on your back with knees easily hanging over the chest; lightly wrap your hands around the knees.

- Let the knees gently open as far as they do easily on the in-breath, with the arms opening outwards from the heart space above the chest as the hands release from the knees, to the side, slightly lower than shoulder height, maintaining the slight curve of the arms, a true sense of opening out from the sternum along the clavicles and the length and power of the arms as they open and resting the backs of the hands lightly on the floor at the end of the breath. Do not engage the lower back, feel it release softly against the floor.

- On the out-breath, the knees float easily toward the chest as the arms gently curve back up and encircle them. Do not consciously engage the abdominal muscles – this work is about release from 'working' the muscles.

- Continue and stay with the exercise for at least three minutes or so; if you need to take a break, you can let the feet rest on the floor, and just move the arms, continuing the focus deep in your centre. When you feel rested have another go.

- Once the rhythm and ease of the exercise have been established, add voice (mmm, f, s, how, etc.) on the return of the knees to the chest as you breathe out.

Title: A Sufi Exercise (from Morwenna Rowe, Voice Practitioner)

Aim: This exercise promotes deep centreing with the movement impetus from the belly, focus, connection to the earth and a sense of inner space. It involves a sequence of three alternate gestures of the right and left leg and arm, with palm of hand returning to resting on the abdomen (belly) coupled with an open 'hah' vocalization. This can last anywhere between 5 and 20 minutes and is most satisfying done in a large enough space for a group working together.

- Start from a grounded position, feet firmly planted heels together, toes angled gently outwards, knees softly bent throughout, spine long, shoulders relaxed; and hands pressing/cupping the abdomen/navel.

- To the rhythm of the recorded drum beat (or work in silence and keep an even rhythm), gesture right leg forward to the floor, extending the foot in front but keeping the knees soft and keeping the weight in the supporting leg and at the same time extend right arm to just under shoulder height, keeping the hand open, allowing a rich, open 'hah' to be vocalized from your centre as the right foot lands.

- Return to centre, foot to starting position and hands back on the belly.

- Repeat with left leg, extending left arm, allowing the same rich, open 'hah' to sound as left foot lands on the floor.

- Come back to centre.

- The sequence continues with a gesture of the right leg to the side, left leg to the side.

- The sequence concludes with the right leg gesturing to the back making sure that the supporting foot pivots slightly inwards towards the direction, whilst maintaining the openness of the belly, groin and inner thighs but preventing the knee from twisting in the endeavour to take the leg behind and then the same with the left, each gesture of the leg and arm followed by a return to centre.

- The entire sequence starts again and continues.

Throughout the exercise the eyes follow the direction of the moving hand. The rhythm is repetitive and even, but the music to which this is performed allows for ebb and flow of energy and speeds up gradually so that you can feel that inner build of excitement, but which throughout, remains contained by the form. There is always a sense with work like this that you have personally been on an enormous journey, which needs still time after for reflection and rest.

BIBLIOGRAPHY

Abram, D. (1997) *The Spell of the Sensuous*. New York: Vintage Books.

Barba, E. and Savarese, N. (1991) 'The Secret Art of the Performer'. *A Dictionary of Theatre Anthropology*. London and New York: Routledge.

Bainbridge Cohen, B. (1997) *Sensing, Feeling and Action*. Northampton: Contact Editions.

Bartenieff, I. and Lewis, D. (1997) *Body Movement: Coping with the Environment*. New York: Routledge.

Harders, Jake. (2005) 'Correspondence.' London: Central School of Speech and Drama. Email. 19 April.

Pert, C. (1997) *Molecules of Emotion: The Scientific Basis Behind Mind-Body Medicine*. New York: Simon and Schuster Inc.

Roth, G. (1995) *Maps to Ecstasy*. UK: Thorsons.

CHAPTER 12

Breath, Theatrical Authenticity and the Healing Arts

RENA COOK

To be inspired – with words, song, dance or art of any kind – is to breathe in, to swim in, to merge with the Muse…becoming totally yourself.

Joy Gardner-Gordon (Gardner-Gordon 1993, p. 7)

Breathing is both the easiest and hardest task to be mastered by the voice user. Bringing the authentic self to the task challenges any voice user daily, be it performing on the stage, in front of the camera, in the boardroom, or before the judge and jury.

Two common assertions form the foundations of vocal development, whether it be speech in the professional arenas or voice for clear interpersonal communication. First, breath is a cornerstone of the free and released voice. Second, breath gives wings to the authentic creative impulse. These fundamentals are so widely held that many voice users, be they teachers, speakers, lawyers, politicians, or performers, may be guilty of giving them a shorter shrift than they demand, a place of lesser importance in the training and development process. In order to re-examine these tenets, to re-affirm why and how breath is taught and studied, how it relates to authenticity and creative inspiration we can look beyond the boundaries of contemporary 'how to' manuals to the writings of numerous Healing Arts practitioners.

I am defining authenticity as the honest presence of the self, simple, pure, without artifice or posturing, without defence or masking. I am including creative inspiration in this discussion as it is crucial to success, not just in the arts as we may typically think, but in all types of interactions. Fresh ideas, innovations, spontaneous and open interactions all happen when we are in the creative state. Voice is added to this triangle as it is the tangible pathway for communication of ideas and feelings to be shared. Breath is the common denominator that not only links authenticity, creative inspiration and the vocal effectiveness but allows them to happen at all.

In the literature of the Healing Arts, breath is frequently described as a master key to healing; the link between the body, the mind and the imagination; the junction between the conscious and the unconscious. If, as many of us agree, the essential ingredient for authenticity is tapping into the unconscious imagination, then it stands to reason that the breath can be our conscious conduit to the unconscious creative state. Taking this assertion still further, breath allows the speaker to stay honest and true in the moment, the voice to remain resonant and expressive, and the body supple and responsive.

I began testing these fundamental truths through the first 20 years of my career as a theatre director and acting teacher, and again more recently as a voice trainer in both the theatre and the corporate world as well. Numerous questions guide my investigations. What constitutes authenticity? How does breath physically, chemically and emotionally so affect the entire human system? How can it be taught effectively and, more importantly, how can it be taken to the interpersonal or public arena and positively affect the outcome of communication? What makes one speaker utterly compelling to an audience and another speaker unengaging? And what role does breath play in this equation? In her book *Finding Your Voice*, Barbara Houseman seeks an answer to this question when she writes, 'The ability to be truly connected and then communicate with clarity and authenticity is universal... Good performers reach the audience, fully convincing and engaging them in action' (2002, p. xiv). From the perspective of the movement trainer, Lorna Marshall, in *The Body Speaks*, believes that

> you must be able to bring your body into free and easy contact with the emotions, other performers, the language of the text, style of presentation and, eventually, the audience. It must be fully alive, in dialogue with your inner life and be able to vividly express a chosen human reality. (Marshall 2002, p. 9)

Is the breath the link that integrates all these necessary and diverse qualities? Through reading, observation and practical application I have attempted to discover clearer explanations, methodologies, strategies and teaching techniques in order to assist the voice user to connect more deeply and consistently to breath that empowers the voice and leads to an authentic impulse.

Gay Hendricks, in his audiotape entitled *The Art of Breathing and Centering*, describes breath as the meeting ground, 'the healing splint' between the conscious and the unconscious, the connective tissue as it were. If, as some performance philosophies teach, the unconscious mind yields more spontaneity, more honesty than does the conscious mind, then it stands that the more a voice user delves into and activates the breath, the more creative and authentic choices the unconscious yields. The dialogue with the inner life can be deepened and enriched through attention and focus on the breath.

In addressing the awakening of the unconscious, Dennis Lewis, in his book *The Tao of Natural Breathing* writes, 'To breathe fully is to live fully, to manifest the full range and power of our inborn potential...unleashes the energies of life' providing 'pathway(s) into the deepest recesses of our being' (1997, p. 17). The voice user then, through deep and deliberate breath practice, can release a wider range of intuitive, creative choices. She can tap into power and vitality, having a greater chance of making the journey to the deepest recesses of the soul and sharing its contents with the intended audience.

If 'superficial breathing ensures a superficial experience of ourselves', then superficial breathing leads to superficial performance (p. 15). Lewis asserts that 'breathing is a living metaphor for understanding how to expand our narrow sense of ourselves' (p. 27). To broaden the range of choices available, to expose new ways of acting and reacting, speaking and moving, the voice user, or the communicator, must position breath work at the centre of the discipline. Mediocre performance is peppered with a narrow, limited range of choices stemming from voice users who don't know themselves or the world they inhabit. It is through the study and practice of deep breathing that we can 'experience for ourselves how the alchemical substances of matter and the magical ideas of mind are linked in the unified, transformative dance' (p. 22).

Hendricks also asserts that breathing is a metaphor for life. Full inhalation and exhalation is giving and receiving fully. The in-breath can be equated with the willingness to experience life fully, while the out-breath is willingness to express the self completely (Hendricks 1989). 'Giving and receiving' are common images used in communication theory, often defining the communicator's task as taking in what others send out and giving back voice and action in return. It follows then that the in-breath is what the voice user takes in or receives and how they are affected by that information. The out-breath is what the voice user says and does in response to what they have received. If a deep and fully realized breath is not present, the authentic voice cannot speak, the spontaneous creative moment is stilled.

The theoretical and practical crossover between the healing breath and the communication breath is becoming more common. Such notable practitioners as Kristin Linklater and Catherine Fitzmaurice base much of their esteemed voice and acting work on ancient Eastern practices of yoga and tai chi. In her book *Freeing the Natural Voice*, Linklater acknowledges the growing interest in these disciplines to 'free the emotional and psychological self' (1976, p. 4). Fitzmaurice, in an article entitled 'Breath is Meaning', reveals that she began studying yoga in 1971. She found that yoga stretches, coupled with bioenergetic tremors, help the actor achieve 'a fully relaxed torso' (Hampton and Acker 1997, p. 249).

In his book *Full Catastrophe Living*, John Kabat-Zinn acknowledges the performance breath in support of his argument encouraging the necessity of the healing breath when he says, 'All professionals who make special use of their breathing as part of their work, such as opera singers, wind-instrument players, dancers, actors, and martial artists, know the value of breathing' (1990, p. 52). He writes,

> We will have to train ourselves to attend to a process (the breath) that not only cycles and flows but that also responds to our emotional state by changing its rhythm, sometimes quite dramatically... Tuning in to it brings us right into the here and now. It immediately anchors our awareness in the body, in a fundamental, rhythmic, flowing life process. (Kabat-Zinn 1990, p. 49)

Kabat-Zinn's choice of the word 'anchor' is a useful image for the voice user who, in the midst of performance or presentation, while fighting many factors vying for attention – self consciousness, monitoring, rustles in the audience, a bungled word or sentence – must learn to focus and re-focus attention on the breath. It anchors the performer to the moment. When concentration must be the purest, it is the breath that provides the surest and most direct link to the artistic impulse, the moment of truth. 'This (breath) is an extremely effective way of locating a peaceful center within yourself. It enhances the overall stability of your mind' (Kabat-Zinn 1990, p. 53). At a time when the voice user longs for a peaceful centre, fear and self-doubt tear at the fabric of honest word and action. It is in these moments when the well-practised link to breath can be the most valuable. For without the calming, stabilizing force of the breath, the authentic artistic moment is gone.

In *The Tao of Natural Breathing*, Dennis Lewis asserts: 'The process of breathing, if we can begin to understand it in relation to the whole of life, shows us the way to let go of the old and to open to the new' (1997, p. 25). One of the primary focuses of voice and movement training is to remove tension habits, old ways of speaking and moving, thereby releasing fresh modes of expression. Through the practice of regular deep, abdominal breathing the voice user can allow the body, voice and imagination to be open to new and more creative choices.

Kabat-Zinn also speaks to the breath's transformative power to open creative options as he states,

> When we are mindful of our breathing, it helps us to calm the body and the mind. Then we are able to be aware of our thoughts and feelings with a greater degree of calmness and with a more discerning eye. We are able to see things more clearly and with a larger perspective... And with this awareness comes a feeling of having more room to move, of having more options, of being free to choose effective and appropriate responses. (Kabat-Zinn 1990, p. 56)

How often, as communicators, as voice users, have we sought a greater sense of inner space, more creative options in our physical and vocal expression? We acknowledge the need for, or are encouraged to 'make choices' and then wonder why the choices made are predictable and limited. Choices made without an awareness of or openness to breath will always be thin and uninteresting. On the other hand, choices that are rooted in breath, that come from the centre and are grounded in breath, will have space, life and authenticity. As Kabat-Zinn observes, 'when we systematically bring awareness to the breath and sustain it for extended periods... with it comes a growing sense of the breath as a dependable ally' (1990, p. 56).

In my personal practice of late, a growing understanding of the breath as being both conscious and unconscious, and the active link to the autonomic nervous system, has inspired a change in the way in which I approach the breath, voice and my teaching. According to Dr Andrew Weil, the Director of Integrated Medicine at the University of Arizona, in his book *Breath: The Master Key to Self-Healing*, the breath is the only system in the body which is both conscious and unconscious. Two sets of muscles and nerves can each operate the system fully. Breath is the only function with which you can control the involuntary nervous system. The involuntary nervous system, also called the autonomic nervous system, is made up of the sympathetic and parasympathetic systems. The sympathetic system prepares the body for emergency, fight or flight, by speeding up the heart rate, raising the blood pressure, diverting blood away from the surface of the body; breath becomes shallow. Those of us who work in front of audiences of any kind know this set of symptoms as stage fright or performance anxiety. The parasympathetic system has the opposite effect on the body; it slows heart rate, lowers blood pressure and deepens the breath. The two systems normally work in tandem with a flow back and forth appropriate to the situation. Most of us, with our schedules as hectic, stressful and chaotic as they tend to stay, live with these two systems out of balance, the sympathetic system working overtime to the detriment of our health and our creative impulses. Once the sympathetic nervous system is engaged, access to the creative impulse or the authentic voice can be denied. Breath work goes to the heart of this imbalance. And as breath is the only part of the equation that is conscious and voluntary, it is the key to consistent access to the unconscious where the artistic, creative spirit resides.

With these understandings of the breath, a systematic approach to the training emerges, a synthesis from various sources in both the healing worlds and voice and movement practice. I have invited my students along on this journey, practising various exercises, rearranging elements, lengthening, shortening, soliciting their feedback and encouraging them to help me draw conclusions. Our collaboration has proved enriching not only for me but for them as well. I see the results in their bodies, hear the results in their voices; they notice changes in themselves and each other. They are able to articulate what processes enhance breath, the authenticity of impulse and the creative state.

EXERCISES

Title: Resonating energy centres (adapted from an exercise called 'Toning the Chakras' by Joy Gardner-Gordon).

Aim: To centre the breath, encourage vocal vibrations and open the body's receptivity to vocal resonance, I have adapted an exercise originally intended to open and tune the charkras.

How often: This exercise can be done daily or several times a week. It generally takes ten minutes to engage with it fully.

Where: Any quiet space.

- In an easily erect seated position, focus on the tail bone area (the first chakra) and intone the vowel 'eh', on a comfortably low pitch. With continued focus on the tailbone, add an image of the colour red, as if red vibrations move the sound into and spinning out of the tailbone. Repeat each sound at least five times.

- The focus of attention then moves to the space between the navel and the pubic bone (the second chakra), the sound is 'o', the pitch may move slightly higher. The colour orange is used to inspire vibrations into and spinning out of the abdominal area. Strengthen the vibrations, feel that space come to life from the energy of the sound vibrations.

- Next the focus of attention moves to between the navel and the sternum (the third chakra). The sound is 'ow', the colour is yellow, pitch again moves naturally up a tone. Feel vibrations of yellow sound move to and spin out of this area.

- The focus now moves to the chest (the heart or fourth chakra). The sound is 'ha', the colour is green. Feel vibrations of green sound move through the chest, lungs and heart. Make that area alive with your sound vibrations.

- Shift the focus to the throat and mouth area (the fifth chakra), the sound is 'oo', the colour is blue. Feel the area come alive with vibrations as the colour blue spins though it. Adjust pitch up if your voice feels the need.

- The forehead now becomes the focus (the sixth chakra) and the sound is a hum, the colour is indigo, the pitch may need to move up a tone. Imagine that the vibrations are streaming out of the forehead. Drill indigo sound vibrations out through your forehead.

- The final energy centre is the top of the head (the seven or crown chakra), the sound 'ee' helps to move vibrations into that area, pitch is comfortably higher. That colour is violet. Feel the violet sound vibrations spin out the top of head, imagine a long stream all the way to the sky.

Each sound is repeated five times or so. The various pitches may cover an octave or smaller depending on what feels comfortable for your voice on any given day.

As a conclusion to this exercise, vocalize with an easy glide on any of the above sounds from the tailbone through the top of the head and back again several times. A roll up the spine will get you to your feet. Try a few sentences from a speech, presentation or memorized poem to see if the body is more receptive to the vibrations of the voice, the pitch freer, the sound more released, the breath more deeply rooted in the body.

Title: Running breath energy (adapted from an exercise called 'Microcosmic Orbit' by Mantak Chia, (Chia and Chia 1993), pp. 269, 335, 431).

Aim: This exercise is intended to energize, focus attention, stretch the depth of the breath and brings attention to the upward direction of alignment. The over-riding image of this exercise is inhaling up the back of the body and exhaling down the front.

How often: This exercise can be done daily or several times a week.

Where: This can be done in any quiet space, seated or standing.

- The first step is to place attention on major body energy centres: starting with the tailbone, moving to the kidneys, the centre of the back opposite the heart, the top of the thoracic spine, the base of the skull, the top of the head, forehead, mouth/throat, heart, sternum, navel and back to the tailbone. Spend a few moments at each spot, breathing with the image that the breath can stimulate vibrations.

• Then starting from the tailbone, let the inhale travel up the back through each point to the top of the head. Next the exhale travels down the front of the body, through each energy centre, the exhale taking the form of a gentle 'fff'. This circular breath is repeated five to ten times.

• By adding humming on the exhale, then opening on an 'ah' glide, followed by 'oo', and 'eee' this breath-energy exercise can open resonance. Some students have commented that it also relieves vocal fatigue.

Title:	Grounding with dowel rods
Aim:	This exercise is intended to energize the breath and grounding the feet in preparing the voice for speaking.
How often:	Do this exercise before each presentation or performance.
Where:	This exercise can be done in any quiet space. For this exercise you will need a dowel rod ½ to ¾ inch in diameter, approximately 36 inches in length (these can be found in hardware stores).

• In bare feet, allow toes to hang over the rod, breathing deeply, softening jaw and tongue, thinking a long easy spine.

• Slowly walk across the dowel rod, lingering for a count of ten at toes, ball of the foot, two places in the arch and the heel, surrendering to any discomfort until feet are flat on the floor once more. For variety you can exhale on an 'sh' or 'v' and breathe out a sign of relief as you move to the next point on the foot, or even vocalize on an easy 'ha ha ma ha ha'. These are distractions from the discomfort of the exercise and provide an opportunity to easily begin the warm-up of the voice.

• When you step off, be aware of what is different in the feet, the knees, the hips, lower back, top of head, jaw, shoulders, breath. I find a pre- and post-test very enlightening. Check the sense of feet against the floor, place of breath, feeling of balance before walking across the rod. Contrasting changes in the body after the walk usually stimulates much conversation.

Title:	Dowel rod for breath and resonance
	This three-part exercise is based on a tai chi sequence (adapted from an exercise devised by David Carey).
Aim:	This exercise is intended to deepen the breath and encourage vocal resonance.

- Holding your dowel rod gently in hands with arms down and shoulders soft, lift rod to chest height as breath flows in. Extend hands/arms straight back down on the exhale.

- Bring rod back to chest on the next inhale, then extend arms straight out in front on exhale and down to starting position.

- Finally bring the rod up on the inhale all the way over the head, then forward in an arc on the exhale.

- Sounding begins with a hum on the exhalations for several full sequences, then opens to an 'ah', finally to any vowel, any pitch.

Conclusion: we breathe between 15,000 and 20,000 breaths in a 24-hour period or 100 million in a lifetime. If we can increase the efficiency of each breath by only 5 per cent, by the end of the day we will have increased the efficiency of our bodies a thousand-fold. 'If you can learn to breathe even a little bit better, you will notice immediate, profound shifts in your physical, mental and emotional well-being' (Hendricks 1995, p. 4). Breathing deeply into the body releases barriers that block creativity. Authentic, conscious, abdominal breathing increases our ability to handle a higher charge of energy, as if plugged into a universal socket, we radiate from within. As communicators we can then connect to voice, language and finally action, commanding the audience's attention, compelling them to be present, to hear and to be forever changed.

BIBLIOGRAPHY

Carey, David (1999, 2000) Vocal skills class taken at the Central School of Speech and Drama, London, England.

Chia, Mantak and Chia, Maneewan (1993) *Awaken Healing Light of the Tao.* New York: Healing Tao.

Farhi, Donna (1996) *The Breathing Book.* New York: Henry Holt and Company.

Fried, Robert (1999) *Breathe Well, Be Well.* New York: John Wiley and Sons, Incorporated.

Gardener-Gordon, Joy (1993) *The Healing Voice.* California: The Crossing Press.

Green, Debbie and Rowe, Morweena (1999, 2000) Movement class taken at the Central School of Speech and Drama, London, England.

Hampton, Marion and Acker, Barbara (1997) *The Vocal Vision: Views on Voice.* New York: Applause Books.

Hendricks, Gay (1989) *The Art of Breathing and Centering* (Audiocassette). New York: Audio Renaissance.

Hendricks, Gay (1995) *Conscious Breathing.* New York: Bantam Books.

Houseman, Barbara (2002) *Finding Your Voice.* London: Nick Hern Books.

Kabat-Zinn, Jon (1990) *Full Catastrophe Living.* New York: Dell Publishing.

Kayes, Gillyanne (2000) *Singing and the Actor*. London: A&C Black.

Lewis, Dennis (1997) *The Tao of Natural Breathing*. California: Mountain Wind Publishing.

Linklater, Kristin (1976) *Freeing the Natural Voice*. New York: Drama Book Publishers.

Marshall, Lorna (2002) *The Body Speaks*. New York: Palgrave Macmillan.

Rama, Swami and Ballentine, Rudolph and Hymes, Alan (1979) *Science of Breath: A Practical Guide*. Pennsylvania: The Himalayan Institute Press.

Sellers-Young, Barbara (2001) *Breathing, Movement, Exploration*. New York: Applause Theatre and Cinema Books.

Speads, Carola (1992) *Ways to Better Breathing*. Vermont: Healing Arts Press.

Weil Andrew (1995) *Spontaneous Healing*. New York: Ballantine Books.

Weil Andrew (1999) *Breathing: The Master Key to Self Healing*. Massachusetts: Thorne Communications.

Zi, Nancy (1994) *The Art of Breathing*. California: Vivi Company.

SECTION 4

Breath and Performance

JANE BOSTON AND RENA COOK

The following five chapters all trace their critical and practical origins to the performance training traditions of the West as they have been exercised over the past century. In a range of stylistic approaches, these authors utilize a mix of historical and reflective practitioner research models to articulate their accounts. Many of the authors make parallels with other spheres of social and cultural significance where pedagogical strategies are shown to be useful to a wide range of voice users not only on the stage but in other professions as well. By so doing, they draw attention to the differences that the application of breathing skills can make within performance and which can also be adopted by those in other arenas to great and lasting effect. In tracing various training objectives for the breath and investigating some of the assumptions about training values, as can be seen elsewhere in this collection, intriguing philosophical questions are also raised about the paradoxes inherent in actually training the breath in the first place.

Starting with David Carey, who outlines the history of breath within voice training in the British conservatoire over the past century, there is a thorough explication of the foundational processes that have emerged over this period, with a specific account of relevant exercises that utilize a range of breathing approaches and are then applied to the expression of the voice.

Jane Boston offers an account of breath from her stance within the British conservatoire as a voice practitioner and provides an example of a workshop process in which the practical and metaphorical uses of breath can provide students with a method for fully embracing work with heightened verse. Breath in this context provides a bridge between the authorial voice, involving the formalism of Romantic verse, and the knowable sensations of the body and poetics of the student themselves. In this way the structures of language that may have appeared at a distance from the roots of emotion are mediated by the revelations provided by the breath in the individual body and provide, thereby, the student with alternative but equally meaningful sensations of language itself.

As an actress and a teacher situated within the North American conservatoire, Lisa Wilson follows with an account of her career trajectory in the field, supplemented by teaching case studies in which 'common' issues about breath are worked through with examples of how to effectively approach them. This gives the reader invaluable insight into the ways in which practitioner reflection evolves over time to generate new positions about 'received' ways of working.

Using the sources of Laban Movement Analysis and approaches from the Indonesian Amerta Movement work, Dr Katya Bloom outlines the work she does in helping students to recognize their own movement vocabularies and habits, as well as to increase their confidence, extend their range and release their creativity. She looks at the significance of psychotherapeutic concepts in adding to current understanding about movement training for actors and in defining the importance of breath as part of a more therapeutic movement model. She notes how this opens up enormous possibilities for breath in the moving body to be understood both psychologically and physically.

This is complemented by a personal account from Judylee Vivier who vividly documents her artistic and pedagogical journey towards her current position training graduates in the North American conservatoires. She draws attention to the subtle processes involved in the art of inhabiting the position of voice practitioner, acknowledging that the filtering of influences experienced from other practitioners in tandem with those acquired through politics and culture are indispensable in shaping the role. Central to her pedagogy is the transformative possibilities of the breath, enabling deeper teaching sensibilities and revealing an expanded humanity for teacher, student and audience alike.

CHAPTER 13

Transformation and the Actor

The responsive breath

DAVID CAREY

Have you ever considered the connection between thought and breath? How the clearer your thinking is, the more deeply you breathe? When I began work on this chapter, at first my thoughts were unfocused and I noticed that my breathing was quite shallow as my mind shifted from one idea to another. As my thoughts became more lucid, however, my breathing became deeper and more centred. My body and mind were so coordinated that as I became inspired mentally, my body responded with physiological inspiration: the flow of breath and the flow of thoughts were in complete association.

It is a connection that we perhaps take for granted, so let me examine this association further. Our breath is closely related to all the elements of our humanity: to our innate life-regulating system; to our instinctive and learned emotional responses, to our internal and external environment; and to our psychic responses to those environments, such as intuitions, inspirations and thoughts. Breath is vegetative, emotive, intuitive and expressive. It is thus deeply involved in our integrated psycho-physical totality.

Each in-breath we take is a response to one or all of the following: the physical impulse which arises as a result of chemical messages received by the brain that the body is in need of an oxygen/carbon-dioxide exchange; the psychic impulse which arises from the desire to give form to an inchoate thought; and, the psycho-physical impulse which arises from the need to express an emotion. Each out-breath is, therefore, the physical release of excess CO_2 into the atmosphere and simultaneously the potential expression of thought or feeling. Each out-breath is the concrete effect of these internal events in the external world. Thus, inspiration is both the physical act of inhaling air; and it is creative motivation. Expiration is both the physical act of exhaling breath; and, it is transitive expression.

Consequently, to stop breathing as a human being is literally to die. And to hold one's breath as an actor causes the character to die metaphorically: to stop thinking and feeling; to stop expressing. The in-breath enables us to conceive, the out-breath enables us to express. This is the fundamental nature of the relationship between breath and mind. In our psycho-physical reality breath is intimately connected to both our physical and psychic selves. And it is, therefore, at the core of the actor's being, their skill, art and craft, as thus:

- The actor is a human being with his/her own emotional, psychic and physiological history.

- The actor is a skilled performer who has learned to adapt his/her vocal and physical habits in order to create a range of characters whose social and personal lives may be very different from the actor's own.

- The actor is an expressive artist who is able to transform him/herself imaginatively in order to respond creatively in the moment as the character.

- The actor is a craftsperson who uses his/her knowledge of language, human behaviour, emotional reality and theatre process to develop dramatic and engaging storytelling.

To fulfil these roles of human being, performer, artist and craftsperson the actor must breathe, fully and deeply, at one with the character and him/herself.

And yet as human beings with our own emotional, psychic and physiological history we have developed habitual patterns of behaviour that feel safe, right, natural and real. If we try to alter these patterns of behaviour, we may feel unsafe, wrong, unnatural and false. Many of these behavioural patterns concern how we breathe – how we breathe for life, how we breathe to speak, how we breathe when we listen, how we breathe in different emotional states.

If the actor in training is to expand psycho-physically to meet the characters he/she plays, that actor must be able to acknowledge his/her own patterns of breathing, recognize those which are healthy and supportive, and work to re-pattern those which are unhealthy and unhelpful. Thus the actor develops a breathing system that is responsive to the full range of expressive impulses of character, thought and feeling.

The actor in rehearsal, if he/she is to transform psycho-physically into a particular character, must be open to the breathing patterns of that character as they are manifested in the rhythms of thought and in the dynamics of emotion within the play's language. Actors need to be able to use their breathing systems creatively in order to meet the challenges of both characterization and performance.

The actor who fails to develop a responsive breathing system, or fails to use that system creatively, reduces a character or performance to his/her own behavioural habits. They do not expand or transform – they diminish and play safe.

What, then, makes for a responsive psycho-physical breathing system? To answer this question, I shall trace the development of breath in actor training over the last century to arrive at an overview of current practice.

For at least 50 years from the founding of the first modern drama schools at the beginning of the twentieth century, most British actors were encouraged to learn a system of breathing known as 'rib-reserve'. 'Rib-reserve' is described most fully in J. Clifford Turner's classic text *Voice and Speech in the Theatre*. Following exercises to develop breath control through training the diaphragm and intercostal muscles, he proceeds to describe the 'final form of control' in which the lungs are first expanded by simultaneous expansion of the rib cage and lowering of the diaphragm. Turner further explains,

> Breath is then exhaled by raising the diaphragm, but when this has taken place the ribs are not allowed to descend but remain extended. The diaphragm is then contracted to replenish the breath supply and again is allowed to rise to expel a quantity of breath. Breath is alternately inhaled and exhaled by the diaphragm which contracts and relaxes rhythmically... This is sometimes found to be difficult but, with perseverance, ultimately becomes as simple and easy as breathing in any other way. (1956, p. 17)

The term 'rib-reserve' seems to have originated with Dr W. A. Aikin, who was Turner's teacher at the Central School of Speech and Drama (founded in 1906 by Elsie Fogerty and Sir Frank Benson). In 1912 Fogerty was introduced to Dr Aikin, who had recently published his practical book on voice, *The Voice* (1900 and 1910), in which he set out the anatomical and phonetic principles of voice and speech production. Fogerty quickly recruited Aikin to her staff, where he remained for over twenty years, contributing immensely to the formation of the Central ethos that was to be passed on to such acolytes as Turner and Gwynneth Thurburn, who both trained at Central shortly after the First World War.

Aikin promoted 'central' (or intercostal-diaphragmatic) breathing, which focused on expansion of the ribs surrounding the solar plexus and contraction of the diaphragm as far as it affected the upper abdominal wall. This was in contrast to other forms of breathing, which concentrated on either a purely costal or a lower abdominal breath and which were seen as unhealthy at the time. He also advocated rib-reserve breathing for performance purposes – that is, the maintenance of an expanded chest throughout a speech or song (specifically, according to Aikin, a lateral expansion at the level of the sixth and seventh ribs) while breathing diaphragmatically. Fogerty (in *Speech Craft*, 1930), Thurburn (in *Voice and Speech*, 1939) and Turner all promote central breathing, but interestingly it only seems to be Turner who follows the full rib-reserve approach. Both Fogerty and Thurburn prefer to relax the ribs at the end of each breath rather than maintain their expansion. Whether this indicates a male/female distinction in their pedagogy is not clear.

However, in the last 50 years, a more natural, less prescriptive approach to breathing has developed. While this new approach maintains elements of the previous system – such as the engagement of both intercostal and diaphragmatic activity – it has also embraced influences from bodywork practices such as Alexander Technique as well as from Eastern meditative traditions and martial arts training in order to create a system which is more integrated with the body's functioning as a whole. Its evolution can be seen in the writings of practitioners such as Cicely Berry, Arthur Lessac, Kristin Linklater and later, Patsy Rodenburg .

In particular, both Berry and Linklater were concerned with finding 'the essential truth of (the) voice' (Berry 1973, p. 15) and felt that rib-reserve helped to produce an unreal or artificial voice, one associated with the heightened acting of an earlier period rather than one which sounded natural and authentic to a modern ear. While both of them encouraged strength and muscularity in the intercostal muscles, it was the focus on the diaphragm and the abdominal muscles that became more important. Berry in *The Actor and the Text* (1987) even notes a development in her own thinking from an upper abdominal focus to a deeper, lower abdominal one that is more in touch with one's feelings.

The emergence of this new approach was partly necessitated by post-war developments in British theatre. With the advent of method acting, the growth of film and television and the interest in kitchen-sink dramas, the 1950s and 1960s produced a cultural revolution in theatre and theatre training that led initially to the rejection of anything false or unnatural. Theatre training began to change as a result.

In particular, an ambivalence about vocal training developed. Those schools which maintained a strong focus on vocal training had to contend with students who saw no relevance in it to their future employment. Other schools watered down the amount of technical work on the voice. And others simply threw the baby out with the bathwater, rejecting any form of training as false or unnecessary. It was into this environment that Berry's *Voice and the Actor* (1973) and Linklater's *Freeing the Natural Voice* (1976) were published. In these books, the authors provided systems for training the voice which were couched in terms that were more accessible to the contemporary generation of actors and thus were able to lay the foundation for a fresh approach which paid full attention to the development of technical skills in the context of the development of a modern artistic sensibility.

With respect to breath, Berry and Linklater emphasized that breath is connected to thought and intention rather than to performance style. This insight enabled voice teachers to focus training on the need to develop a form of breathing which felt more authentic because it was related to the body's impulses and was responsive to the demands of character and text: a responsive breathing system.

A RESPONSIVE BREATHING SYSTEM

Let us again ask the questions: What makes for a responsive breathing system? And how can one use it creatively?

I would suggest that in current practice a responsive breathing system is one which enables the actor's voice to respond flexibly to the demands of different performance contexts. The foundation of this ability lies in the breath: in its centre, capacity, sustainability and support. All four of these components or attributes of breath are necessary for a completely responsive system.

Centre: a word that is widely used in actor training but which can often be mysterious to students. A group of acting students recently asked me what 'centre' was. When I explained that humans have a literal centre of gravity inside the abdominal cavity, a number of pennies seemed to drop. Envisaging an internal centre enabled them to find a deeper sense of connection to their breathing and voices. I relate this 'centre' to the T'an T'ien of T'ai Chi – an internal focus of energy from which action flows. I also conceive of it as the core of our will and emotions – as it seems to me that these live more in our bellies than in our hearts or mind. Once our breath connects to this centre (that is, once we align our breathing fully with our life energy, will and emotions) the voice gains an audible strength and authenticity.

Capacity: total human lung capacity averages seven litres, while normal tidal volume (the amount of air we exchange simply for vegetative purposes) is only 0.5 litres. While it is possible to phonate using only tidal air, humans normally increase their respiratory intake to two or three litres for speech purposes. This augmentation in volume is achieved by increasing the expansion of the lungs. Although the lungs can potentially be increased in three directions – vertically, laterally and anterio-posteriorally – optimal expansion is achieved by employing the first two options only, since the latter tends to restrict the vertical and lateral potential. Vertical expansion is the most effective means and is most healthily achieved through contracting the diaphragm downwards into the abdominal cavity and simultaneously relaxing the abdominal muscles to allow for the displacement of the abdominal contents. The lowering of the diaphragm draws the lungs down, so causing them to inflate with air. It is the vertical expansion that connects the physical activity of breathing to 'centre.' Lateral expansion is principally achieved through contracting the external intercostal muscles, which act to raise the ribs outwards and upwards. This action of the ribs, to which the lungs are attached, causes the lungs to expand outwards, again causing them to inflate with air.

Sustainability: for the human voice to maintain sound it requires a confident supply and steady flow of air from the lungs. The confident supply comes from having inhaled enough air for the purpose of speech and this is achieved by the effectiveness of vertical and lateral expansion. However, increasing lung capacity requires contraction of a number of muscles that, if they were to simply relax, would cause a rapid deflation of the lungs. Expanding the ribcage causes it to lift slightly in opposition to gravity; suddenly relaxing the muscles which lift the ribcage allows gravity to exert its influence again. As the ribcage expands, the ribs also twist slightly; suddenly relaxing the muscles allows them to recoil quickly. These forces need to be resisted if the flow of air is to be maintained in a steady and sustained way. It is by slowly relaxing the inspiratory muscles, in particular the intercostal muscles, that we can achieve this sustainable flow of air. This sustaining power of the intercostals is an important attribute. In particular, it enables the speaker to maintain the flow of thought energy with confidence, rather than having to interrupt this flow in order to take a breath. But on its own it may not provide emotional depth to the voice or facilitate dynamic changes of intensity or pitch. For these, support is necessary.

Support: for the human voice to achieve different intensities of sound it requires a means whereby the pressure of air from the lungs can be varied. This variation in pressure can be achieved in two main ways: by changing resistance to the flow of air within the larynx and by changing the exhalatory pressure being exerted on the lungs by the muscles of expiration. While small changes in intra-laryngeal resistance may be appropriate at times, particularly for singers, excessive laryngeal constriction is potentially damaging to vocal health – sudden or sustained high intensity sound produced in this way can lead to hoarseness and, ultimately, vocal nodules. Increasing vocal intensity, in my view, is more optimally achieved by first increasing breath support; that is, by increasing the activity of the muscles of expiration that can exert exhalatory pressure on the lungs. The muscles that are particularly appropriate for doing this are the abdominal muscles, especially the internal and external obliques and the transversus. Contraction of these muscles exerts an upward pressure on the diaphragm. When we breathe out, the diaphragm relaxes upwards into the thoracic cavity causing exhalatory pressure to build up underneath the lungs. The contraction of the abdominal muscles can raise this exhalatory pressure by causing the abdominal contents to push the diaphragm up into the thoracic cavity with more force than its own relaxation pressure will create. Increasing or decreasing this support of the abdominal muscles will thus contribute to variations in vocal intensity. Here again we have a connection to the abdominal centre. So both in terms of inspiration and expiration establishing a strong connection to centre, an integrated and responsive respiratory system is enabled. However, just as the sustaining power of the intercostals on its own may be insufficient for all expressive purposes, so too may the sole use of abdominal support. While it gives a strong emotional impetus to the voice, it may not provide enough sustaining capacity to manage the flow of thought energy with enough forward momentum or flexibility. It is when the system acts as a dynamic whole in conjunction with energized intentions and not just as discrete constituent elements, that the actor will have the scope to make creative expressive choices. When these choices become available, the actor will communicate thought and feeling in active relation to character and situation rather than with passive respect to the actor's habitual behaviour.

So, what does it mean for the system to work as a dynamic whole? For the actor, ideally the thought/feeling impulse instigates the process of inspiration. The neurological inspiration initiates the physical inspiration that is executed by the muscles of the diaphragm and the external intercostals. The expansion of the thoracic cavity increases lung capacity, drawing sufficient air into the body to enable phonation to take place. The relaxation of these inspiratory muscles initiates exhalation. But for sustained and supported vocal sound, the full relaxation pressure of these muscles must be resisted in order to manage the flow of breath in an efficient and consistent way. If, after we had breathed in, we simply let the muscles relax, our breath would rush out in a sighing sound that would rapidly decrease in pitch and volume. However, if our aim were to produce a sustained hum or vowel sound of a steady pitch and volume, the difference in intention would lead to an altered function in the respiratory musculature. This would entail the controlled relaxation of the intercostals together with an increasing involvement of the abdominal muscles of support. Variations in thought and feeling translate partially into variations of breath flow and pressure, which in turn influence the expressive values of intensity and pitch. This integrated process requires a subtle and precise marriage of intention and technical skill.

The actor in training, therefore, needs to develop an awareness of and control over his/her respiratory musculature in order to establish a strong foundation for the integration of technical skill with the acting process. The acting process alone – however detailed the actor's research and investigation of thought and feeling might be – is not necessarily sufficient to be able to sustain vocal vibration and adjust intensities of sound in order to shape the vocal performance of text for the listener's ear. Therefore, work on breath must make the student-actor aware of his/her process of and capacity for breath. Thus he/she can learn to manage it in a way that allows the system to be artistically responsive to the thought/feeling impulse while being alert to the shaping possibilities of the out-breath in expressing that thought/feeling. This should enable the student-actor to grow in his/her awareness of the restrictions that habitual patterns impose on his/her expressivity and to develop the possibilities of new patterns of breathing which are capable of extending that expressivity to encompass dramatic characterizations that are outside his/her everyday experience.

This process will entail progressing through a number of stages of training: work on releasing the breath from old habits that restrict the development of a fuller capacity; muscular work on the diaphragm, intercostals and abdominals in order to develop their vigour and flexibility; conscious work on connecting the breath to the thought/feeling impulse; and, expressive work on applying breath to the shaping of text in different performance contexts. The professional actor in performance then needs to be able to link respiratory activity with imaginative intention and emotional impulse to create a psycho-physical whole that will communicate effectively with both his/her fellow actors and with the audience.

I recently worked with an experienced actor who was having difficulty finding enough breath to sustain him through a scene in a production that had been playing for several weeks. He recognized that his breath was placed too high – that is, he wasn't connected to the centre. By giving him the opportunity to experience a freer, more centred breath as the character outside of performance, I was able to set him on the path to a fuller realization of the character in performance. This illustrates how essential it is for the working actor to stay connected to his/her training and how easy it is for other professional demands to over-ride the creative process. Although this actor had created a real character – one full of vitality and presence – through his application of acting process, the fact that he was experiencing some technical difficulty reveals the need to integrate this acting process fully and consciously with a responsive respiratory system.

Yes, he is a skilled performer who can adapt his vocal and physical habits in order to create a character whose social and personal life is very different from his own. And he is an expressive artist who is able to transform himself imaginatively in order to inhabit his character fully as a human being in his own right. And he is a craftsperson who uses his knowledge of language, human behaviour, emotional reality and theatre process to develop dramatic and engaging storytelling. But it was because he is a human being with his own emotional, psychic and physiological history that he was experiencing difficulty in performance. As a human being he had been 'holding his breath' in rehearsal – out of fear, anxiety and ambition – and this had bled into his characterization and then into his performance. Through troubleshooting his problem with breath, he discovered the need to breathe fully and deeply, at one with the character and himself.

EXERCISES

Title: Inspirational response (this exercise is a development of one that I originally learned from Meribeth Bunch Dayme)

Aim: The aim of this exercise is to enable you to initiate voice with ease, using your natural breathing cycle. It can be used at the beginning of a daily vocal workout and is best done in a good resonant room with few distractions.

- Find a chair which is firm enough to support your sitting bones but not so hard that you will become restless. The chair should also be of a height where your feet can easily touch the floor and where your thighs can be parallel with the floor.

- Sit on the chair so that your weight is evenly spread across your posterior, your spine is long and your hands are resting gently on top of your thighs. Relax your face, your shoulders and your mind.

- Now begin to pay attention to your own natural breath cycle. Try not to alter how you are breathing; just notice how your body moves as you breathe in and out.

- Now let your attention focus on the moment where the in-breath changes to the out-breath. Notice the sensation as the body changes from one type of activity to another. Notice where is the deepest point in your torso that you can feel this happening.

- Keep focusing on this moment of change and on this deepest point in the torso. Now, mark this moment of change from in-breath to out-breath with a little sound – 'huh' – think of the sound coming from that deepest point in the torso. It can be quite a quiet sound to begin with, just enough voice that you can hear it.

- Repeat this several times until you become more familiar with the sensations. Now think of making a stronger commitment to the sound so that it gets slightly louder. Again, repeat this several times. Now let the sound begin to lengthen out more, so that it sounds like a sigh. You're still focused on the moment of change from in-breath to out-breath, but now you're using more of your breath to mark that moment. Perhaps you're breathing gets deeper too. Just let your body respond to the simple demands you're placing on it.

- After you have repeated this long sighing 'hu-u-u-uh' sound several times, let it change into a long 'ha-a-a-ah' sound that you are sustaining on a single note. This will sound like you're almost singing.

- As you become more confident with this, let each fresh in-breath change into a different sustained note. You can also vary the vowel sound that you're sustaining. Play with these changes for a minute or so and then let your attention focus on your breath cycle again. Has it changed since the beginning of the exercise? If so, how?

- Bring the exercise to a close. How do you feel?

Title:	Paired rib-reserve (this exercise is based on J. Clifford Turner's approach to rib-reserve training in *Voice and Speech in the Theatre*.)
Aim:	The aim of this exercise is to enable you to develop an awareness of rib-reserve breathing. Rib-reserve breathing is essentially a performance-level activity – it is not expected that one would employ it as a breath-for-life activity or even in breath-for-everyday-speech. Mastering rib-reserve takes time and should not be undertaken by beginners. It is best done in a classroom setting under a teacher's supervision.

- Find a partner and have him/her stand in front of you, but facing away. Help your partner find an aligned, relaxed stance with feet about hip-width apart and weight evenly distributed across both feet.

- Locate the approximate position of your partner's sixth and seventh ribs at the side of the rib-cage. You can do this by finding the bottom of the breastbone

– rib seven attaches to the sternum at this point. By moving your hands to a position horizontal with the tip of the breastbone at the side of the rib-cage, you can take hold of their ribs approximately at the level of ribs six and seven.

- With the fingers of each hand wrapped around the ribs on either side of your partner, let your thumbs point across their back towards the spine. Let your partner guide you to a contact that gives him/her a firm sense of pressure without constriction. Make sure your partner's shoulders are relaxed.

- Your partner should first breathe out fully and then, as he/she breathes in, think of filling his/her lungs on either side underneath your hands. You should be able to feel your partner's ribs move outwards from the spine in a lateral direction as they do so. Your partner should then breathe out easily but fully, letting the ribs return to their rest position. Continue with several cycles of breathing. You may feel more movement on one side than the other – this may happen if your partner habitually breathes more with one lung than the other. Encourage your partner to think of breathing evenly with both lungs, expanding the ribs equally on both sides, but don't worry if he/she finds this difficult to begin with. Discourage any tendency to lift the shoulders or breastbone.

- As your partner becomes more familiar with this lateral expansion and release of the rib-cage, help him/her to regulate the movement by counting in the following way: Breathe in 1–2–3; breathe out 1–2–3–4–5–6. If he/she can breathe out for longer than a count of 6, then you can increase the count to 8 or 10, but there should be no attempt to make the breath last beyond what is comfortable.

- Once your partner is comfortable and confident with the movement of the ribs, ask him/her to place one of his/her own hands on his/her upper abdominal wall (the epigastrium) so that he/she can observe the movement here as he/she breathes in and out. This movement occurs as a result of the downward movement of the diaphragm. If your partner has difficulty feeling anything, encourage him/her to think of filling down into the bottom of the lungs as he/she breathes in and of blowing the air out as he/she breathes out.

- Having felt these two movements – the ribs and the diaphragm – separately, it's time to bring them together. Ask your partner to keep a hand on the epigastrium while you return to holding their ribs. Ensure that your partner's shoulders are relaxed and that he/she is standing in a relaxed, aligned position. You're going to start counting again, but this time when you count '1', your partner should breathe in with a focus on expanding the rib-cage; when you say '2', your partner should continue to breathe in, but this time lowering the diaphragm; and on '3', he or she should breathe out slowly and easily for a mental count of 10 or 12, letting the ribs release and the diaphragm relax at the same time. It helps to isolate the movement of the ribs and diaphragm on the in-breath in this way to begin with, but the ultimate goal is to do them simultaneously.

- So, once your partner is comfortable and confident with the previous exercise, ask him/her to keep his/her hand on his/her epigastrium while you hold his/her ribs. You're going to count again, but this time when you count '1', your partner should breathe in, expanding the rib-cage and lowering the diaphragm at the same time; on '2', he or she should begin to breathe out slowly and easily by letting the diaphragm relax for a mental count of 6 or 8; and on '3', your partner should continue to breathe out, but this time letting the rib-cage release for a mental count of 6 or 8. To isolate the movement of the diaphragm and the ribs on the out-breath in this way prepares for the activity required for rib-reserve breathing.

- To engage rib-reserve breathing, therefore, first ensure that your partner is comfortable and confident with the previous exercise. Ensure that his/her shoulders are relaxed and that he/she is standing in a relaxed, aligned position. Once again, ask your partner to keep a hand on his/her epigastrium while you hold his/her ribs. You're going to count again, but this time when you count '1', your partner should breathe in, expanding the rib-cage and lowering the diaphragm at the same time as before; and on '2', he or she should begin to breathe out slowly and easily by letting the diaphragm relax as before for a mental count of 8 or 10; but, instead of letting the ribs release on '3', your partner should keep them elevated while breathing in again by lowering the diaphragm. This may take some practice for your partner to feel comfortable and confident, but the aim is that he or she should be able to continue breathing in this manner – keeping the rib-cage expanded while inhaling and exhaling through the activity of the diaphragm alone. In this way, a reserve of air can be maintained in the rib-cage for whenever it might be needed in performance.

Title: Spine breathing

Aim: The aim of this exercise is to access a full and responsive breath using imaginative stimuli. It can be used as part of a daily vocal workout and is best done in a good resonant room with few distractions.

- Lie on the floor in a semi-supine position. Make sure your head is supported so that your neck can be long and your forehead is parallel with the ceiling – you may need to place one or two paperbacks under your head to achieve this. Let your hands rest gently on your abdomen with the elbows resting on the floor by your side. Imagine your back lengthening and widening across the floor.

- Become aware of your breathing and, as you breathe in, imagine that your breath is filling up your spine from your tail-bone to the crown of your head. As you breathe out, imagine your breath flowing down the mid-line of your body from your brow to your groin. Let this imaginary journey of breath repeat with each new breath cycle, but try to be very specific in your sensory awareness of the various stages of the journey. Don't forget to let your whole spine fill with breath.

- As you become familiar with this journey, add an 'FFF' sound to your out-breath. Let the 'FFF' sound brush down the front of your body for several breath cycles. Now, change the 'FFF' to 'VVV', imagining the vibrations of the sound tingling down the front of your body for several breath cycles. Then let your lips close together so that you can make an 'MMM' sound. Start to play with the pitch of the sound. Let the pitch of your voice move easily through its range as the vibrations move down your body.

- Now, as you continue to play with your pitch on the 'MMM' sound, let your breathing take care of itself and focus your attention instead on the 'MMM' sound. Imagine the vibrations rolling round your mouth as the pitch moves. Think of moving the pitch up through the range as well as down. After a short while let the vibrations out on a long 'AH' sound – let your jaw drop open and feel the space in your mouth as you imagine the sound pouring out of you. Play with the pitch of the 'AH' sound for a few out-breaths and then change to an 'OO' sound, shaping it with your lips like a fountain. Play with the pitch of the 'OO' fountain for a few out-breaths and then change to an 'EE' sound, letting your lips soften into a smile. After a few out-breaths on 'EE', bring the sound to a close and observe your breathing. Focus your awareness in your rib-cage for a few breaths and notice how it expands as you breathe in and relaxes as you breathe out. Then focus on your abdomen and notice how it also expands and reduces in response to your breath cycle. Although different muscles are acting in different ways at different points in the cycle, the overall feeling is of the body (and lungs) expanding as you breathe in and reducing as you breathe out.

ACKNOWLEDGEMENT

Sections of this chapter were originally developed for *With One Voice*, a one-day workshop for Vocal Process given in collaboration with Gillyanne Kayes (www.vocalprocess.net). My sincere thanks to Gillyanne for her support and encouragement.

BIBLIOGRAPHY

Aikin, W.A. ([1900, 1910] 1950) *The Voice: An Introduction to Practical Phonology*. London: Longmans.

Berry, Cicely ([1973] 2000a) *Voice and the Actor*. London: Virgin.

Berry, Cicely ([1987] 2000b) *The Actor and the Text*. London: Virgin.

Fogerty, Elsie (1930) *Speech Craft: A Manual of Practice in English Speech*. London: Dent.

Lessac, Arthur (1997) *The Use and Training of the Human Voice*. Third Edition. Mountain View: Mayfield.

Linklater, Kristin ([1976] 2006) *Freeing the Natural Voice*. Revised Edition. Hollywood: Drama Publishers.

Rodenburg, Patsy (1997) *The Actor Speaks*. London: Methuen.

Thurburn, Gwynneth (1939) *Voice and Speech*. London: Nisbet.

Turner, J. Clifford ([1956] 2007) *Voice and Speech in the Theatre*. Sixth Edition. Edited by Jane Boston. London: A&C Black.

CHAPTER 14

Breathing the Verse

An examination of breath in contemporary actor training

JANE BOSTON

INTRODUCTION

Central to the curriculum of the training actor is the breath and the way in which it produces artistry. This is not a new thing. According to theatre academic Jacqueline Martin, the relationship between proper breathing and effective speaking was recognized as far back as the ancient Greeks and Romans (Martin 1991, p. 37) The Elizabethans also observed its role in the art of oratory, explained by a teacher at the time as needing to be 'natural and lively in delivery' and flowing 'out of the liquid current of Nature' (Joseph 1964, p. 8).

Subsequently, many of the great twentieth century theorists of acting also acknowledged the place of breath at the heart of their practice. French actor and director Jacques Copeau (1879-1949), for example, had this to say about the centrality of breath in artistic expression: 'A voice which does not breathe becomes dull, collapses on itself and becomes sad. It flounders like someone dying' (Rudlin 2000, p. 66). Constantin Stanislavski, likewise, was quick to critique the actor who failed to harness the potency of an inner energy that he clearly associated with the breath and named inspiration:

Scenic action is the movement from the soul to the body, from the center to the periphery, from the internal to the external, from the thing an actor feels to its physical form. External action on the stage when not inspired, not justified, not called forth by inner activity, is entertaining only for the eyes and ears; it does not penetrate the heart, it has no significance in the life of a human spirit in a role. (Stanislavski 1981, p. 49)

Breath was also central to the acting theories of Antonin Artaud in the first quarter of the twentieth century. He derived these from the Kabbalah where breath is conceptualized as 'the breath of life that God infuses into His creatures' (Benedetti 2005, p. 226). He believed it was possible to influence the soul itself through the conscious working of the breath:

I had the idea of using knowledge of the breath not only in the actor's work but training for the actor's profession. For if the knowledge of breath illumines the colour of the soul, it can even more rouse the soul and allow it to blossom. (Benedetti 2005, p. 227)

This profound relationship between the internal impulse and external expression is pragmatically singled out more than half a century later by leading British theatre practitioner Declan Donnellan. He observes that when the inspirational connection is weak, it can wreck the relationship between the actors and their text: 'When actors do not take in enough breath, they savage their text and butcher the longer thoughts' (Donnellan 2005, p. 156).

Breath's seminal role in the craft of the actor has been similarly situated over the 20-year period that I have been teaching voice and acting in the British acting conservatories. However, although the primacy of breath in training the actor has been widely recognized, I would argue that it has remained an under-theorized area of the work. I would suggest, therefore, that in order to better understand the ways in which breath can help shape the artist and enable their expressive development, the relationship between breath as inspiration and its outer expression as voice needs to be more closely scrutinized in the training studio.

Currently, much of the actor training work on breath has focused upon student achievement of the desirable quantity of breath for each mode of expression. This is clearly important, since optimum levels of breath supply are vital for human health and expression. However, quantity is not the only significant feature of breath. There also needs to be an appreciation of how it enables an individual to integrate his or her own psychophysiology into their artistic expression. In tandem, quantity and quality can foster ever more effective artistic outcomes from the training on a greater range of levels.

In order to further aid these artistic goals, it is clear that a refinement of the manner, terminology, imagery and pace by which a teacher conveys the information and not just the information itself, will require investigation. Ideally, this should take place alongside growing student awareness about the multi-functioning of breath itself so that they can experience a range of profound opportunities for changing old patterns and harnessing new techniques.

But it is most important that students should be encouraged to experience and understand the distinctions between the various functions of breath during the course of their training. It is absolutely crucial that they be able to distinguish between four primary functions of the breath. First is its importance in life-giving metabolic gas exchange, second is its ability to influence the autonomic systems of the body, third is its support for all communication and fourth is as the vehicle for an individual to become more sensitized to deeper textual interpretations. The conscious and unconscious possibilities awakened by experiencing these distinctions will provide the student with valuable and profound opportunities for changing old patterns and harnessing new techniques.

This examination of aspects of vocal pedagogy for the training of the actor in relation to an increased awareness of breath, therefore, has a two-fold aim. First, to render conservatoire training objectives clearer for teacher and student alike and second, to suggest that a deeper sense of individual artistry can be attained when working in a more detailed way with the breath. A colleague at the Royal Academy of Dramatic Art (RADA) recently said, 'Until the breath supports effectively, the artist can never be free' (Moulton 2006, personal communication). This concept will be examined with the aim of enabling it to be more coherently understood within contemporary vocal training programmes.

In the first part of this chapter I examine the significance of breath in relation to interpretive work on verse language, and the growing psychological awareness of the individual. In the second part, I examine a training process that fosters a deeper relationship between the individual, their breath and verse text.

BREATH AND HEIGHTENED VERSE TEXT

Within actor training, one of the principle roles of the breath is to be at the service of the spoken word. Clearly, however, the valuable principles enshrined within these practices are ones to which any student may subscribe who wishes to enhance their connection to the word, written or spoken. As we have seen, contemporary acting theorists from Stanislavski onwards have suggested that any performer's connection will be enhanced when a clear connection is made with an internal physical need that is equated to the impulse of the breath. They have also made a strong case for the importance of relating the communicator's own physiology and psychology to the word in order to render its expression as close as possible to the original impulse or intention of the author.

The conscious application of breath is clearly one of the ways in which to enable a dialogue between interior and exterior and allow the vocal artist to go beneath a superficial interpretation of language to discover deeper psychophysical resonances. It can also help the student to manage the distinction between heightened verse as 'extraordinary' language and 'ordinary' speech. (Heightened verse in the context of this chapter refers to verse forms that possess an abundance of metaphor, richness of vocabulary, poetic conceits, pronounced metre and rhyme, often in highly patterned visual and auditory ways.)

Breath and interiority

Movement therapist, Katya Bloom suggests that we can partly attribute the interiority of actor training philosophies to the wider human psychological drive to bring the disjointed parts of the self back together. In mirroring the 'depressive position' (Bloom 2006, p. 52–3), as described in the psychoanalytic theory of Melanie Klein, this drive refers to a wish for wholeness of body and mind often alluded to in contemporary voice and acting work. It is a journey that has psychological as well as physiological consequences:

> The implied softening of the defensive processes that keep parts separate would seem to suggest a relaxation of the body, both the neuro-musculature and the breathing, an acceptance of one's relationship to gravity and an ability to tolerate the mixture of feelings and sensations constituting one's own inner depths. (Bloom 2006, p. 52–3)

Of particular interest in the link Bloom makes between mind and body, is the qualitative difference fostered by the breath as the body and mind becomes less defensive. This mirrors instruction in wider acting curricula where students are invited to become less defensive and more genuinely self-knowing in order to create the conditions for conscious transformation later in the training. For Bloom and also for leading voice theorist Kristin Linklater, defensiveness can be the enemy of the artist: 'Defensive neuromuscular programming develops habits of mind and muscle that cut us off from the instinctual connection between emotions and breath' (Linklater 2006, p. 22).

Language and the symbolic space

Alice Oswald, in the 2005 Ted Hughes memorial lecture, observed that poets such as Hughes (former UK Poet Laureate) write in order to give fuller life to 'the creatures behind the language ... the raw animal truth underneath, the truth of gesture and intonation' (Oswald 2005). These 'creatures' can be regarded as symbolic representations of the feelings behind the utterance of language and are what the performer can hope to connect with through the breath.

The communication of language can be rendered functional and shallow if there is no ability to access these layers of symbolic thought. The interpretive student, therefore, may find that their ability to harness the breath will allow them greater opportunity to contact these symbolic levels and enable the communication to be even 'wider and richer than human language', involving 'the whole sacred and speechless background of nature' (Oswald 2005). This too, will provide a link to all poetic writing past and present in which is found a 'feeling for syllable and rhythm, penetrating far below the conscious levels of thought and feeling, invigorating every word; sinking to the most primitive and forgotten' (Eliot 1966). It will also encourage the practice of thinking about language at a level that goes beyond the cliché commonly heard in today's public relations minded society that renders it as a mechanistic tool. The language of poetry, as we have seen, however, is entirely different:

> In our own language verbal sounds are organically linked to the vast system of root-meanings and related associations, deep in the subsoil of psychological life, beyond our immediate awareness or conscious manipulation. It is the distinction of poetry to create strong patterns in these hidden meanings as well as in the clearly audible sounds. (Hughes and Heaney 1997, p. 568)

In stark contrast to this, contemporary society has organized itself (albeit unconsciously) not only to split the body from the mind and the word from the body, the spontaneous impulse from the secondary impulse, but also everyday discourse from the richness of these oral roots. As the task of the vocal interpreter is to function beyond all linear limitations, it is clear they must be encouraged, through training practices, to encounter holistic, exceptional and transformational experiences with language. Only when these opportunities are made available, can active pleasure be taken in sounding language aloud as it vibrates through the body on the breath, allowing the word to make contact and trigger individualized sensations. By remaining in balance and by not inappropriately binding the musculature of the body, the possibilities for feeling language as a physical sensation can be made that much more available.

Pedagogical precedents

It has long been accepted in vocal pedagogy, that in order for the word to be worked off the page for performance purposes, a variety of practical strategies need to be exercised. The former 'twentieth century practice of reading literary texts silently... eliminated the possibility of experiencing (its) music' (Martin 1991, p. 33). As a consequence, practices in voice training, particularly in the UK, have been designed to overcome the silent internalization of language in favour of its live oral expression where a richer auditory life can reveal the intentions of the writer.

Speech neuro-biology has recently revealed more about the complexities involved in separating the component parts of language. This highlights the challenges faced by performers as they move from reading, which is a more left hemisphere based activity, to the prosodic activities of speech and intonation that are more influenced by the right hemisphere (Karpf 2006, p. 58). Scientists have shown, for example, that: 'the brain takes speech and separates it into words and 'melody' – the varying intonation in speech that reveals mood, gender and so on. (S)tudies suggest words are then shunted over to the left temporal lobe for processing, while the melody is channelled to the right side of the brain, a region more stimulated by music' (Sample 2004, p. 9).

These studies suggest that future practical strategies devised to connect performers with language should be ever more sensitively designed in the light of the knowledge that the brain has to work on several levels at once in order to handle sound, tune, rhythm and meaning. Because breath is so intimately linked to the production of sound, it can be a significant factor in enabling these sophisticated processes to work at optimum levels. Whilst individuals are very obviously 'programmed' to respond readily to speech in the primary auditory cortex of the brain, '(we) perceive it almost obligatorily' (Sample 2004, p. 9), it is harder work to attach this conditioned response to a deeper understanding of the tune, image and rhythm of language, in order to reap rich communicative outcomes. The reward of embodied speech, it seems, will only fully come when the breath can be utilized as a means of connecting with an individual performer's emotional and physical life:

> Because of the direct and uninterrupted connection with the breath source, vowels can be directly connected with emotion, but only if the breath source is as deep as the diaphragm. The solar plexus is knit into the fibre of the diaphragm and is the primary emotional receiving and transmitting nerve centre. (Linklater 1992, p.16)

Coupled with diaphragmatic awareness must be also that of the transversus muscles as they provide not only a functionally reliable place to speak from but one that is deeply connected to the 'geometric centre' of the body. (Catherine Fitzmaurice at her July London Workshop 2007.) For the performer who has to ensure that the words they read on the page must, when spoken, come authentically and spontaneously from their mouths, an awareness of this responsive and reflexive breathing musculature will be, therefore, crucial.

As is the case with many teaching approaches, learning occurs most effectively when there is significant value attached to allowing the body to respond actively to the sensations of language. In making the link between the reflexive breath musculature, resonance and conducted vibration, the breath shifts the word from its place simply as print and is returned to the realm of the human experience in the body; in synthesizing somatic knowledge with intellectual knowledge, in this manner, the beginning of a genuine embodiment of the word can begin to occur.

A breath and voice process designed to generate a balance between heightened literary verse on the page and a contemporary spoken ownership can be found in the following account of a voice and text workshop held over a three-day period during the London International Workshop Festival in November 2004. Reference will also be made to subsequent workshops at the Voice and Speech Trainers Association (VASTA) in the summer of 2005 and RADA in January 2007.

A POETICS OF BREATH AND THE ROMANTIC POETS

In the middle of the twentieth century, American poet Charles Olsen wrote an influential essay about the use and interpretation of poetry in which he located breath as the bedrock for his new poetics:

> Verse now, 1950, if it is to go ahead, if it is to be of essential use, must, I take it, catch up and put into itself certain laws and possibilities of the breath, of the breathing of the man who writes. (Allen 1960, p. 386)

Olsen considered that the more an individual writer could contact their breath and locate it as a source of communicative energy, the more engaged with their own experience their writing would become. He regarded breath as providing the key to a new poetic voice which was influenced less by an external aesthetic and more from within through the breath of authorial sensation, composed of 'energy transferred from where the poet got it' (Allen 1960, p.387).

In a similar way, breath can be utilized as the starting point for an experiential process of learning in which the richly imaginative and emotionally volatile worlds of the British Romantic poets in the eighteenth and nineteenth centuries can be accessed. In this process the link with Olsen's thesis is maintained but applied differently and the focus is shifted from the poet to the interpretive stance taken about the poet's work by the modern performance student, who can sometimes find that the Romantic poets are inaccessible. It is argued that by the utilization of their psychophysiology on the breath, a creative link to the mind and emotion of these writers can be made. In this way the breath both facilitates the authentic voice of the writer, as in Olsen's aesthetic, and that of the student interpreter.

What follows is a guide to this process that can be adopted by anyone who reads or who is interested in the spoken word, as a speaker or as an interpreter, and it will provide a means to access the primary intention of any spoken text. It is aimed at the student who will work through this in the ideal context of a group situation but for the student who is on his or her own, the work will also be equally applicable.

Olsen's argument stems from his position that in breath there is a return to the origin of human proportion – a place that is rooted in being and not separated or distant from that which is involved in being human. In his view, breath can provide the core sensation from which to produce language and if re-traced can also provide the map back to the thought that produced it in the first place. In other words, breath can provide the return to the impulse as much as it can also provide the means to re-experience the original impulses. Being in touch with the breath allows each individual to stay in connection with the body from where 'all act springs' (Allen 1960, p. 397).

The process of enabling an entry into the state of a poem's inception by intuiting the early impulses of its creation by means of the breath has, then, to be amongst the first of the interpreters' tasks. This relates to concepts defined within psychoanalytic theory that help to link the creativity of the reader to an ability to come afresh to something that has already been created. It is intended that this can begin to mirror the delight taken by the poet in penning the poem in the first place, termed by the poet Carole Satyamurti (after the psychoanalyst Winnicott) as a 'first time every quality...like discovering a room with new objects in it, which I could explore and rearrange as I liked' (Satyamurti 2003, 1960, p. 39). By creating this kind of psychophysical space with the breath, the intense pleasures of the early childhood experience can be mirrored and the possibility of a real connection between reader and author can be made.

It is important that each individual who wishes to discover for her or himself the culturally valued writing of the past, should be able to do so without the burden of the anxieties that can often be experienced when facing such work. If any negative hangovers remain from early educational experiences with poetry, for example, it becomes crucial to counteract them.

At the outset of the process, a calming focus on the simple movement of the breath at rest can begin to enable a more open and easeful approach to any first reading. Metaphor, too, can help to provide the mental and physical conditions for entry into the creative state, provided here by the notion of setting forth, as in the embarkation of the protagonist in Byron's early poem *Childe Harold's Pilgrimage, Canto III*. In this poem, for example, the literal leaving of the land for a sea voyage puts us in mind of the first early steps we all take away from maternal presence towards self-discovery and links us, too, with a view expressed by Stanislavski, in which the communicative journey is likened to something that radiates outwards and where experience gained is likened to an inhalation back into the body:

> Influenced by Yoga, Stanislavski imagines communication as the transmitting and receiving of rays of energy much like psychic radio waves. Our breathing puts us in touch with these rays. With every exhalation, we send rays out into the environment and with every inhalation we receive energy back into our bodies. (Carnicke 2000, pp. 20–1)

The workshop

By starting with a reading of the description of the protagonist's journey in *Childe Harold* by Byron, with its strong rhyme and rich vocabulary, the reader/listener is provided with an experience of writing that seeks to create vivid and active pictures about a sea journey driven by the breath of a storm.

The preparation for listening is an important stage in this interpretive process. An invitation must be made for the mind to be cleared in order to receive the variety of sound pattern and imagery in the verse and temporarily stem the insistence of everyday speech to which, as we have seen, we are only too readily programmed. Following on from this, the physical contact provided by a shake out around the body, allows for the release of superficial tension and an exploration of the ribs and a process of stretching provides a crucial tactile element to the process. It is vital that the mind and the body work together so that the mind in body and body in mind connections are always present. The sequence is as follows:

1. Hold the ribs of a partner (or your own if no partner is present) to feel their expansion and to understand their movement in multi-dimensional ways, including the subtle anterior to posterior diameter of the upper chest in relation to the lateral expansion of the lower ribs.

2. Play the ribs as if they are a squeezebox by drawing them out sideways on their elastic and sprung energy and move them accordingly. This reinforces the swing of the lower ribs away from the body and provides an energetic focus for the lateral expansion of the lower ribs. Overall, this is part of a long process of ensuring that the ribs become sensitized to the active process of the inhalation of the breath and to the fact that they must also fall back to a place of rest after the breath has exhaled. This will then allow the body to utilize the most effective muscles for the support of the out- breath in the form of the transversus abdominal muscles and will not rely on any unproductive squeezing of the ribs themselves. (Notes on the transversus muscles gratefully acknowledged from the Catherine Fitzmaurice workshop, London, 16–20 July 2007)

3. Grasp own ribs tightly, as if fingers were as a corset within which the breath can work to expand beyond the hold, to experience their flexibility. Then, turn knuckles inwards towards the ribs and imagine that the elbows pointing to each side of the walls of the room you are standing in are able to have extensive lateral reach as a result of the inflation provided by the rib swing, giving the added impulse of an assertive mental action to the movement.

4. Stretch the ribs when doing side-bends, sending one arm at a time towards the ceiling and gently over the side of the head laterally, leaving the free arm to pat the intercostal muscles between the ribs on the stretched side, as if patting a full bodied pony on its flank. This offers a sense of the dimension of space between the ribs that can link to the possibilities of an increased volume of air in the lungs and an enhanced sense of literal inspiration.

5. Lie down on one side with a hand placed on the upper most side of the ribs and that same elbow directed towards the ceiling, with the aim of moving the ribs towards the ceiling in order to counter the collapsing effects of gravity. This is one of the most immediately tangible exercises for sensing what the ribs can do when asked to really move. It can also aid the sensation of elastic recoil, as the breath naturally returns to the body after a vacuum has been created by its departure and provides a strong sensation of how the thoracic anatomy functions. (I first experienced this at a Kristin Linklater workshop early in the 1990s.)

These exercises help to provide an alert physical state where self-consciousness can fade and ones own moment-to-moment presence can be registered.

This is to be followed with work influenced by leading European physical the-atre practitioner Patricia Bardi, in which participants can connect with each other by tuning into their own breathing rhythms. As very quickly breathing patterns within any group are imitated, this can provide a useful starting point for gathering a group together for united purposes or finding your focus as a solo participant.

Seat yourselves in a circle and mirror the breathing patterns around you and then focus in on your own breath and let the opening and closing of your palm resting face up on the top of your thighs mirror this movement, like a flower. Let the breath influence the movement rather than the other way around. Then take in your sur-roundings with your eyes and think about your own breath and theirs as distinct and as it can also join together. Use the idea of letting a sound arise on the breath that you can turn into a sustained and sung tone and see if you can finds ways of join-ing your sound with others around you or of varying your pitch from theirs in har-mony or disharmony as you choose. Finally, focus on the Laban influenced manner of moving around the space in which different paces (fast or slow), direct or indirect trajectory, horizontal or vertical planes of movement and eye contact with each other (or not), can be experienced.

Continue, then, with more Patricia Bardi-inspired exercises, using pair work to communicate to each other across the space, connecting to making shapes and mir-roring each other and finally adding sound. Initially this can be done with abstract sound and then it can be followed with words from a list of verbs and nouns ex-tracted from the poem by Byron. These words can be explored and connected to in a way that is similar to an approach Kristin Linklater has made widely accessible in her published works. By placing these words (on paper) around the space in clusters we can call a 'psychic pool of language', comprised of 'the senses, the emotions, memory, personal association, imagination and vowel and consonant dynamics' (Linklater 1992, p.40), the aim is to access both an emotional and a visceral response to the language as you explore.

Next, with your own paper to hand, is the invitation to write your imaginative and emotional responses to the verse you have just experienced with the stipulation that the writing should be free and associative and begin with the line:

'I set off for places unkown'

British poet and creative writing tutor Peter Sansom calls this process 'hot-penning – the mainstay of any writing workshop' and it works well in any practical context to free the mind for focused acts of creativity. Finally, it is important to read your words out loud as a means of generating a conscious bridge between the emotional compass of the Romantic writers and your own experiences and to feel the 'taste' of the language in your own mouth.

Having literally embarked on this 'journey', it is then important to embrace the idea of the exploration or discovery that can take place along the way and to keep at bay any internal forces of discouragement (Sansom 1994, p. 41). Since discovery can also lead the individual towards conflict, an inevitable part of the creative process, this part of the workshop is designed so that participants can encounter the kind of sensations leading movement theorist Gabrielle Roth (Roth and Loudon 1989) offers in her Five Rhythms work, where staccato is the rhythm she equates with conflict and an acknowledgment of it can be extremely fruitful.

Roth's Five Rhythms work provides a way to experience psycho-muscular energy in a 'managed' state of anger and conflict that can also provide a way of connecting the diaphragm to a direct expression of these emotions as language. (Conflict, for example, can be located on the diaphragm as a sharp action, with a sharp beginning and an end using the punctuation of the out-breath on HA.) These staccato sensations allow the breath to work hard and then to release in relation to the action of the diaphragm. Continuing in this vein, utilize the widely documented Linklater panting of the out-breath on Ha, mentally focused at the top of the double-domed muscle of the diaphragm, followed by faster panting and then a final palpitation or flutter to really get the focus of the breath into the musculature and experience a strong sense of physical relationship to an assertive breath.

Once the concept of staccato breath has been located it can then be combined with the idea of flow to provide a mirroring of the state of the chaos of adolescence as conceived by Roth, to set the psycho-physical context for Shelley's poem, 'Ode to the West Wind' (Oxford Anthology 1973, p. 447). The combination of flow and staccato links to Roth's concepts of adolescent turbulence, resistance and emotional volatility and is an extremely useful touchstone for the emotions contained in Shelley's poem.

This practical work provides a crucial muscle memory focus that can be retained whilst the text is returned to in detail. Faced now with potential issues of comprehension and interpretation of both form and content, the universal elements, as theorized by the contemporary Israeli born actor trainer Moni Yakim, can provide an appropriate way to create a non-intellectual entry into the physical and the imaginative world contained within the poem in keeping with an experientially informed process (Yakim, Broadman and Adler 1990):

> An element is. A storm does not rage. It exists. Rain does not weep. It exists.
> The sun does not smile. It exists… When you become an element you have

complete freedom that cannot be experienced any other way. You have no obligation to be of a specific form, to move in a particular way, to make any prescribed sounds. You are free to be the element as you feel it, to do what the element would do, as you are impelled. (Yakim 1990, pp. 90–1)

Consider, then, one of the elements of cloud, fire, darkness, thunder, ocean or volcano and surrender to the way it makes you feel. Lie down on the floor in a comfortable semi-supine position with knees up towards the ceiling and let your mind wander and 'summon all your faculties and focus… Concentrate to where your personal consciousness almost vanishes and your entire being fuses with your (element)' (Yakim 1990, p. 92). After you have spent several minutes with this activity, for at least a minimum of ten minutes, produce an associated list of words about that state of feeling and then write down statements on the page as if you are living that element in a series of 'I am' word association phrases. By so doing, you are beginning to experience something of the psychological landscape of Shelley's poem from the standpoint of your own psycho-physical knowledge.

The process is an imaginative one designed to enable you to mentally and physically surrender to the elemental powers of nature whilst also allowing you to recognize the characteristics of the human condition located in them. In the act of adopting these universal elements, the concept of mentally straining to inhabit the poet's bigger idea becomes lessened and you are able to give recognition to the emotional terrain within. In finding the 'I am' of the element, the 'I feel' of the element and the 'I do' as the element in words, there can begin a genuine process of undoing the analytical brain and engaging with your own responses in relation to given external literary stimuli.

The workshop closure

Following on from the first and second stages of setting out and discovering the territory of the poem, the third and last phase of the workshop is underpinned by the work of Donna Farhi, a leading Yoga and breath teacher, who draws attention to exercises that ask individuals to consider the breath as moving them rather than as something that can be manipulated. In Farhi's approach, an individual's movement is seen to intimately connect with the inspiration of breath. As the body can be moved by the breath, so the mind can be moved by the consciousness of breath as it is drawn into the body, thus helping to draw attention to all the elements involved in staying present mentally and physically in this encounter with language.

This focus on the significance of breath and presence is a component part of the process of ending the workshop. Taking time to breathe out a sigh of relief, as an act of cleansing and releasing and then utilizing the whispered ah, stemming from the Alexander Technique (see Chapter 3, p.52) is to be followed by tactile work on the ribs and curling through a breathing spine, where the giggles, laughter, yawns and sighs that can ensue, help to wipe the analytical canvas and usher in more intuitive responses. With the physical system thus engaged, and the canvas free, it is timely to engage again with the Roth rhythms work, particularly to the lyric phase that she parallels with the emotion of joy. In this way her work provides a physical sensation for the last phase of the journey towards arrival. Taking individually chosen words from the Shelley passage, follow the image of jelly on a plate and move your feet to gain a sensation of the movement of the lyric phase and skip upwards into the space with the language unencumbered by the analytical mind.

At this stage, with the left-brain seemingly on hold, it is possible to experience a sense of aliveness supported by a spontaneous and flexible breath and reflecting a state of physical and mental ease beyond the speech cortex of the brain. Capitalizing on this atmosphere, without giving too much time for the glaze of formality to return, it is important to now write freely for the last time in the same way as before without taking the pen from the page. Start with the key sentence: 'In the afternoon I came unto a land'… in relation to what you would like to find at the end of this metaphorical and physical journey.

Here, again, the breath can provide the key. Where on one hand it can serve as a means of freeing the body from the sympathetic breathing system, preparing the body for a physical state of emergency, it can also serve to unlock the form and metre of the text if you breathe it as it was written. The act of breathing the fullness of the thought on the page finally enables the word in print to come into full contact with the imagination to create a dynamic synergy of self and author on the voice.

CONCLUSION

It is clear that knowing and utilizing the breath allows for the crossover from speech for life to expressive speech for performance. Breath relates in a critical way to enabling the speech cortex and the right hemisphere to work in tandem with each other in order to unlock the printed word in this way. As more is known about the ways in which the brain functions, breath will undoubtedly prove to be a key element in unlocking how this actual process works. Already, however, evidence of practice has shown that by attending to breath as physics, anatomy and metaphor, it is possible to appreciate how these can collectively provide a series of vital keys to enabling a deepened response to language. As we have seen, when the breath is connected knowingly to language, the word becomes something that is far more profound and primordial than just ordinary speech reality for both speaker and listener. Finally, only the breath can ensure that both the form and intention of the given author is technically served when speaking aloud. By attending to breath, the word is truly given life.

In a society that can easily choose to skim the surface in its quest for the quicker route to the message, it seems ever more important to create conscious relationships in relation to the visceral root of what is being said and to give time so that the breath can be a guide to an enlivened speaking state. It is clear that the strategies of using breath to release the inner life of an individual speaker, can provide not only the means to effectively communicate but also to allow them to physically and emotionally engage with the word in order to render it live, deep and meaningful for a listener.

Embedded in daily practice, these processes offer dynamic and progressive models for both the actor training environment and elsewhere, reminding us that in order to stay in touch with our human potential, the manner of contact we make with the breath needs to be regarded as deeply significant. Since breath is at the very heart of what makes us human and provides, in its relationship to language, a key to the ways in which we understand the world, reveal our feelings and communicate with each other, it stands to reason that we must pay it very particular and urgent attention.

BIBLIOGRAPHY

The Oxford Anthology of English Literature (1973) Vol.11. Oxford: Oxford University Press.

Allen, Donald M. (ed.) (1960) The New American Poetry Everyman Original. New York: Grove Press.

Bardi, Patricia. Courses Postbus. 10847 1001 EV Amsterdam, The Netherlands. Telephone 31(0)612038733. info@patriciabardi.com, www.patriciabardi.com.

Benedetti, Jean (2005) The Art of the Actor. London: Methuen.

Bloom, Katya (2006) The Embodied Self Movement and Psychoanalysis. London: Karnac.

Carnicke, Sharon Marie (2000) 'Stanislavsky's System'. In Alison Hodge (ed.) Twentieth Century Actor Training. London and New York: Routledge.

Donnellan, Declan (2005) The Actor and The Target. London: Nick Hern Books.

Eliot, T.S. James Scully (ed.) (1966) Modern Poets on Modern Poetry. London: Collins, Grove Press.

Hughes, Ted and Seamus Heaney (ed.) (1997) The School Bag. London: Faber and Faber.

Joseph, B.L. (1964) Elizabethan Acting. Oxford: Oxford University Press.

Karpf, Anne (2006) The Human Voice: The Story of a Remarkable Talent. London: Bloomsbury Publishing.

Linklater, Kristin (1992) Freeing Shakespeare's Voice. London: Theatre Communications Group.

Linklater, Kristin (2006) Freeing the Natural Voice. London: Nick Hern Books.

Martin, Jacqueline (1991) *Voice in Modern Theatre*. London and New York: Routledge.

Moulton, Darrell (2006) Conversation. Royal Academy of Dramatic Art: October. London, 3 February.

Oswald, Alice (2005) 'Ted Hughes Memorial Lecture 2005.' *Guardian*, 3 December.

Roth, Gabrielle and Loudon, John (1989) *Maps to Ecstasy: Teachings of an Urban Shaman*. UK: New World Library, Penguin Group.

Rudlin, John (2000) 'Jacques Copeau: The quest for Sincerity'. In Alison Hodge (ed.) *Twentieth Century Acting*. London: Routledge.

Sample, Ian (2004) 'Brain Scan Sheds Light on Secrets of Speech.' *Guardian*, 3 February.

Sansom, Peter (1994) *Writing Poems*. Northumberland: Blood Axe Books Ltd.

Satyamurti, Carole (2003) "First time ever" writing the poem in potential space' In Hamish Canham and Carole Satamurti (eds) *Acquainted with the Night*. London: tavistock Clinic Series, Karnac Books.

Stanislavski, Constantin (1981) *Creating a Role*. London: Eyre Methuen Ltd.

Yakim, Moni, Broadman, M. and Adler, Stella (1990) *Creating a Character: A Physical Approach to Acting*. New York: Applause Theatre Book Publishers.

CHAPTER 15

An Integration of Breath, Body and Mind

LISA WILSON

My work in voice is influenced by the many teachers and methods with whom I have had the good fortune to come in contact. I thank them all. My first voice teacher Sybil Robinson at the University of Wisconsin-Madison, a former student of Iris Warren at the Central School of Speech and Drama, carried with her a well-worn binder of notes, the progressions in voice, that had been handed down to her and that she had refined in more than 20 years of teaching. She gave me permission to breathe and to release emotion on voice and through text. Recognition is also due to the vital and creative teachers in The Voice and Speech Trainers Association (VASTA); their ongoing generosity enriches my teaching daily. Most of us can agree that we have learned from a community of generous teachers; many exercises are handed down generation-to-generation and modified when each individual teacher lets the process flow through their personal filter.

My teaching has become eclectic, as many other approaches became known to me in graduate school and beyond – Arthur Lessac, Kristin Linklater, Cicely Berry and Patsy Rodenburg. This rich and diverse background in a variety of disciplines, techniques and methodologies led me to seek integration. I began to incorporate Laban Effort Analysis, Bartenieff Principles, exercises originated by Alexander and

Feldenkrais, Chekhov's psychological gesture, as well as yoga into the voice and movement training I offered. I attended workshops, processed that material, read extensively and experimented with exercises on my own students. My mission remains to facilitate young actors to blend body, mind and voice through integrated training. It is clear to me now that by drawing from a broad range of techniques most acting problems can be investigated and solved from the point of voice, body and mind.

Traditional acting and voice training has always held that releasing the body and voice from tension is the foundation; but we now know that the actor needs more. Both body and voice must respond to impulse and emotion as well as analytical decisions. The voice must go beyond well-supported freedom. It is now widely held that authentic breath response is the key in conquering body tension, focusing the acting thought, accessing the impulse of text, releasing frozen emotions and freeing a stifled or pushed voice.

My current practice now is fully committed to placing breath at the centre of the curriculum. My students and I are dedicated to examining and exploring the ways that the breath links and aids the body, voice, emotions and mind in various performance and real life situations. When the breath is authentic to the moment – on the impulse of the acting thoughts and emotions – the voice, textual and movement choices can successfully integrate and work together.

AUTHENTIC BREATH: THE SOURCE FOR BODY, VOICE AND MIND INTEGRATION

As I strive to articulate on paper what I do in the classroom I have shared my struggle with my family – three greyhounds, one fat cat, two sons and a husband, as well as numerous students in my life. Balancing my laptop precariously, as I shift versions of this chapter and mounds of notes, I am surrounded by dog-eared, heavily annotated texts, sprouting multi-coloured post-it notes, teaching binders and handouts saved from 30 years of my own classes, and the workshops and intensives which have nourished my teaching life. During the passage of time of this writing, two of my greyhounds had to be put to sleep, a third one joined our family and the fat cat is now 14, one son has graduated from college and the other is getting a driver's license, and my husband has had two heart operations. The constant keeping me centred is my voice-movement-breath practice. My personal voice-movement practice incorporates a daily yoga routine, investigations into body/mind/energy work, ongoing work with other teachers, personal stage performance, as well as recognizing the impact which ageing and life experiences have on my instrument.

Breath is the aspect that unifies much of this practice. I seem to have spent my performance life learning to breathe and finding my authentic breath. The free breath of my animals has served as a wonderful observation point for authentic breath connected to need, usage, emotion, intent and circumstance.

Fundamental principles that guide my work toward body/voice/mind integration can be outlined as follows:

1. *Breath is core* The breath is at the core of all voice and movement work. Authentic breath is the source for thoughts, emotions, sound and movement.

2. *Integration is key* Integration of body/mind/voice is key in acting. All action on stage, whether verbal or physical, must have a purpose and is best executed with a free, integrated and expressive instrument.

3. *Engaged breath* Engaged breath and appropriate body effort are central to all action. Authentic breath facilitates spontaneous response to textual, emotional and performance demands, which allow the creative imagination to function as the autopilot on the plane: riding along, keeping the instrument responsive and on-track in support of an action.

4. *Ongoing work* Therefore work with breath must be ongoing during actor training. The actor must integrate free breath with movement, thought and emotion impulse through every stage of the work.

Breath is the foundation, the gas and the power for all voice work. Restriction of breath inhibits both living and performing. Peggy Hackney, author of *Making Connections*, a text on Bartenieff Movement techniques says: 'Breath is the key to life, movement and rhythm… We breathe automatically, but breath can be influenced by and is reflective of changes in consciousness, feelings and thoughts' (Hackney 2002, p. 51).

Similar convictions are expressed in all of the seminal voice books by Berry, Lessac, Linklater and Rodenburg. Their words mesh with my own history as well as comparative case studies of various undergraduate students to help us understand the challenging journey to free an authentic breath.

My performance life began as a dancer. From the ages of 3 to 14 I studied all dance forms and dreamed I would pursue dance professionally. A sudden growth spurt at 14 derailed my dance ambitions. But the body-breath habits acquired during my dance were strongly embedded – holding in the core, frozen shoulders and strong body armouring (i.e. habitual tense and defensive postures of the body – like armour). I brought these habits with me to acting. I did not breathe freely.

My personal journey to a free and open breath mirrors that of many of my students. As I developed, I breathed just enough to keep from falling over, to allow dance movement in various forms, to speak and to be understood. I 'learned to project' when cast in my first speaking role, at Nashville Children's Theatre, performing to a 300-seat house. My director's coaching to be louder and to change my southern vowel substitutions were well intended, but ultimately added new tensions in jaw and throat. My mind told my body that muscular effort must be the key. I pushed to be heard. The higher the emotional stakes, the more I pushed.

Dance habits, my orthodonture, new body changes, emerging sexuality, lack of training, the intense desire to please and fit in and strong doses of self-criticism imprisoned any chance at free breath. My acting gifts of emotional connection, intellectual understanding, expressive movement, discipline and drive were stifled by my voice. Add in my need to control as expressed through head and neck misalignment, holding, jutting – all of which compounded into terrific tension in my throat. The 'rehabilitated' southern drawl not only tensed my tongue and jaw, but it dissociated me from my mother tongue sounds. I didn't know what an authentic breath was and I was clueless as to how free breath could connect to experiencing emotion and pursuing action.

The greatest gift of my Master of Fine Arts in Acting training was discovering breath and finding my voice. The release that came from breathing opened a new world. I became able to cry and talk at the same time! To shout without locking down! To feel my voice and trust it! This is why I became a voice teacher.

Just as I did, my students struggle to find balance, economy and integration, all of which are necessary to support the body as it breathes in harmony with the size of an idea, the emotion and commitment to an action. I think this estranged relationship with the breath and the body comes partly from fundamental unfamiliarity and dissociation from real bodies. TV, movies, magazines make the average real body unreal. Put the phrase 'body image' into a search engine and you will find a huge number of web sites that deal with body image distortion and the recovery and prevention of eating disorders. The famed movement theorist, Moshé Feldenkrais noticed this phenomenon early in his career when he writes,

> Usually one finds that unsatisfactory functioning carries with it an inadequate or incongruent representation of patterns of action as images in the pupil's mind. Not only can the 'wrong' thing be felt to be 'right' and vice versa, but the image of what is being done differs, sometimes strikingly, from the action actually done. (Rywerant 1983, p. 9)

Most students don't like something about their bodies and dislike of belly, teeth, height etc. can negatively affect usage. Likewise, some of the parts students like best, the six-pack abs or the dance turnout, may in fact be standing in the way of reliable free breath. Most people don't find bodies (or at least their own bodies) to be beautiful, amazing miracles. The love of the body, or at minimum the acceptance of it, is vital for the actor. The body is part of the primary working material of the actor.

The body is an expressive container that sources the breath, houses emotion and instinct and enlivens text. In my experience, I have witnessed profound improvements when tension habits are released and deeper breath connections are allowed to flourish.

In order to show more specifically how integration of body/voice/mind come together in my teaching, I will share several case studies of students – their challenges, our work together and the outcomes.

Case study One

Student A, an academically gifted undergraduate, exemplified how patterns of self-perception affect full body engagement, which in turn inhibited responsive breath, openness for re-patterning perception and the ability to connect to an authentic breath. Trained in dance since an early age, the student had a serious holding pattern in the core abdominal muscles and an overly lifted chest, resulting in breath support difficulty. Ambitious and self-critical, she demonstrated disconnections, self-consciousness and a lack of emotional freedom in performance. In working with release exercises she went to the extreme opposite: releasing all muscular involvement to become a heavy rag. During the spinal zipper, after rolling up from a hanging position, she collapsed in the chest and neck. When not in a dance position, her alignment was angular and off-balance. Gaining access to free breath was a two-year process as she accepted the idea that openness and vulnerability are necessary for an actor. As I observed this student's progress, I was reminded of a quote from Reichian Growth Work, 'Feeling tense becomes part of our continuous background experience, so that full relaxation seems like a threat to our existence, as if we are going to melt and drain away completely' (Totton and Edmondson 1988, p. 6).

Utilizing Growth Work exercises to release holding patterns of the eyes, the waist and the belly, Student A was able to allow her body to become more open and she began to release her habit of effortful movement. Once the effortful quality was released, Student A was more successful in exercises aimed at connecting breath and impulse to sound, becoming more authentic as well.

A visceral connection to sounds and words finally came as we integrated ball play into the scene work. As the game demanded full body engagement, she was able to breathe authentically and freely on impulse while engaged to the text.

Case study Two

Broadcaster A sought private coaching to retrain habits born of external imitation of perceived professional presentation. He was a 55-year-old, long-term on-air evening news local anchor, referred for vocal work by his station manager. He appeared mistrustful and apprehensive during the intake session, fearing for his job. My goals were first to win his trust and second to give him tools he could readily use.

The station manager wanted me to change his speech pattern so that he would 'talk normally'. Broadcaster A exhibited a very stiff neck, leading with the chin and contracting the back of the neck. This pattern was reinforced upon initiation of speech. His sound was pressed with a lack of connection to the breath-thought impulse. The odd word emphasis, noted by his manager, was combined with a falling melody pattern. His posture and movements were rigid.

Following a brief explanation of how the voice works and interacts in the body, we began tension release exercises and simple stretches for the upper body and neck. I encouraged him to think of the breath and sound as arriving at the front of the mouth, taking the focus from the throat. We worked to find an open, silent intake of the breath through the mouth, in preparation for sustained sound.

A devoicing habit was mixed with a pressed sound, his interpretation of 'authority-speak'. Practice with release of breath during the stretches, then progressing into sound on the stretches and intoned sounds with physical follow-through proved very helpful.

He made the discovery that different sounds have different durations, useful when emphasizing key words. He began to understood the concept of 'breathing in the thought' before reading the text on the exhale. I noted that his speech pattern was much better than when improvising or doing memorized text when in reading from the teleprompter. The idea of bringing the thought off the page with the breath and releasing it into sound was new to him, as was the discovery of vibrations in the body and face on sound.

I directed him to touch my hand with his finger on completion of the final sound of the line so that he could experience the concept of landing the sound. I encouraged him to breathe the thought in, release the sound with thought, talk to and not at the teleprompter. We also practised lengthening the important words, to vary his delivery.

At the conclusion of our work, his vocal quality was improved through the reduction of held tension, as was his ability to sustain breath to the end of the thought. Broadcaster A's station manager reported he saw a 90 per cent improvement and was very satisfied.

Case study Three

Law Students A, B and C came to voice training to eliminate ineffectual vocal habits and to discover more effective court behaviours. In assessing these students, I found they needed more time to come into their bodies, release, find breath and feel the sound. They needed to discover grounding to the earth, a relationship with the energy through the feet and a sense of the front of their bodies beyond an awareness of the face alone. The workload required of these law students was relentless and was reflected in their bodily tensions and holding patterns. It was a challenge to dissuade the students of misconceived ideas regarding 'effective habits' and to encourage them to embrace open, tension-free bodies and strong voice/breath connections.

Law Student A liked to 'intimidate' with a puffed chest and jutted chin; his breath and neck were completely cut off from his body. Playful release of sound while tossing tennis balls, in addition to working with heightened awareness of alignment gave him a touchstone of what release feels like. His bluff performance and screaming habits were acquired from being a pit trader on the stock exchange floor. Through the work he was able to identify that this former behaviour was no longer effective. He grew in the belief that an aligned body, an easy and open sound and a use of a variety of vocal tactics would serve him better.

Law Student B spoke with an excessively narrow lateral opening of the mouth. He revealed that he had spent years in high school trying to cover braces on his teeth by keeping a closed mouth. He was most successful in finding release when he smiled. An Arthur Lessac exercise, 'woo, woe, wow,' was very helpful in making active lips and cheeks while using a dropped jaw and open channel.

Law Student C had 'abs of steel' from intense pilates work and a fear of looking fat. Making friends with the belly was goal number one. Utilizing spinal zipper and cat-cow encouraged the breath to move into open sound, allowing the student to develop an awareness of the distinction between the belly and spine. Another key breakthrough occurred while lying face down, breathing and voicing, feeling the breath move the front of the body.

Following the initial breath awareness exercises, we addressed other challenges that law students encounter in their voice journey. A five-step programme of vocal exercises included marking the text for breath and thought, a children's story to help make breath and voice gain expressivity and a poem utilizing breath, voice and intention with a variety of scenarios. We next moved to speaking from notes, a more lawyerly activity, marking breaths, sustaining spontaneous thought and working with a variety of verb tactics with text.

The law students, following the six-week course, showed improvement in voice awareness and skill. I encouraged them to continue the work to achieve lasting change by referencing the required text The Right to Speak by Patsy Rodenburg.

CONCLUSION

In my personal and teaching practice I continue to emphasize breath as the source of the body, voice, mind connection. Though further study alters the specific exercises I may use on a daily basis, the precepts remain the same: 1) authentic breath is the source for all strong acting choices, 2) integration of breath is key to freedom of movement, emotion, voice and text, 3) awareness of engaged responsive breath grounds the actor in the moment and 4) ongoing work with breath is necessary to training and improved quality in life and performance. Whether in the practice of Law, performing onstage or doing a television newscast, breath is the vital link to being present, connected and engaged.

EXERCISES

The exercises that follow are used to establish familiarity with freeing the body in order to make breath possible, or to connect free breath to the acting challenge.

Title: The spinal zipper

Aim: To build kinesthetic awareness of the skeleton for a released alignment, to free inhibitory tension in the spine neck and head that can block the free and released breath.

How often: Can be done daily.

First examine a skeleton or a picture of one along with a copy of the key that identifies the bones. Identify and examine.

Standing with eyes closed look inside and visualize your bones:

- how they stack up

- how they relate to the muscles

- how the thoracic vertebrae stack with cushion and space between

- how the ribs grow out of the vertebrae and are integrated into the muscles inside, between and outside between each rib, in what we will call the rib accordion instead of the cage

- how the top eight come into the sternum, the next two come into each other and how the bottom two are floaters and end without connecting

- how the clavicle hinges from the sternum and comes to the apex of the shoulder

- how the shoulders are suspended above the thorax and can rest easily without tension

- how the blades can live settled into the back and the sternum can lift and float

- how the pelvis has two large shelves over the kidneys, the iliac arch and how the hip bones merge and should be level and are above the head of the femur

- how the pubic bone is knit together in front

- how the sacrum is the joint in the back of the pelvis and has a huge amount of energy and feeling and can have movement

- how the pubic joint in the front of the pelvis, has some flexion but no voluntary movement

- how the iliac arch at the back of the pelvis protects the kidneys

- how the pelvis can be balanced if the tailbone drops

- how the lumbar vertebrae, large and strong, can support the lower body, without tension in the belly – if the pelvis is balanced on the femurs

- how the nerves in the sacrum tingle if you rub them with your knuckles (try it!)

- how the large joints move at the shoulder arm and elbow the femoral joint, the knee (try each one in turn: shoulder, elbow, femoral joint, knee)

- notice how the head balances atop the seven cervical vertebrae

- how the top vertebrae is behind your nose

- how the delicate ankles flex, rotate and how the calcanus of the heel creates a tripod with the bones in the ball of the foot on which you balance

- how the toes can stretch up, then forward and out onto the floor without grabbing the floor and how spreading the feet grounds you and lets the spine reach upward

- how the dropped tailbone, the released knees, the long back, the accordion of the ribs, the free neck all respond to breath.

Now:

- Use your hands to feel your own ribs, thoracic vertebrae, sternum, clavicle, scapulae, pelvis, sacrum, tailbone, sit bones, cervical vertebrae, skull and mandible.

- Play with the rotation of the femoral joints of the hips while standing and then seated.

- Explore the shoulder joints.

- Notice the large open area under between the lower front ribs and the pubic bone/front of the pelvic girdle.

- What will be called the belly, the lower abs – belly button to pubis, before finding support from the inner core, we need release held tension in the lower abs.

- Place your hand thumb on belly button, little finger above pubic joint.

- Now *love the belly* – use your hand to jiggle the belly, palpate the muscles in and out and feel your belly – resistance or freedom of the belly.

- Try making a nice open AAAAHHHH and love the belly.

Order of the zipper

- Begin with a sigh and observe the availability of the body to the breath.

- Standing well – feet under the knees, hips over the knees, shoulders over the hips.

- Shake the shoulders, raise drop lightly.

- Let the head drop by lowering the nose and then rolling the neck with awareness in the cervical vertebrae, observe your breath.

- Feel the head hang from the first thoracic vertebra, observe your breath.

- Release each thoracic vertebra, use your hand to check to see if your belly is helping, jiggle the belly. You will be curved about half way over, observe your breath.

- Release each lumbar vertebrae until the need to fold is great and you can fold at the femoral joint, observe your breath.

- Allow the body to hang upside down, let your knees slightly flex, the tail bone is the 'highest' bone in the body.

- Let the torso bounce gently and sway, check for release. Notice where you feel the breath in your body. Be certain not to hold the breath. Where do you feel it move your body? With a deep sigh, does it reach your lower back, your pelvis, your sphincters?

- Reverse the process. Allowing the knees to lift the quads, which brings the knees back into alignment, influxes them and straightens the thighs, the pelvis rolls under and the tailbone points toward the ground.

- Allow the vertebrae of the lumbar area to 'restack' one by one. Checking with a free hand that the belly is not clinching to lift the torso, rather the bones are restacking the body without assistance from the abs. Notice your breath.

- Allow the thoracic vertebrae to restack one by one, feel the shoulder blades slide back into place sliding down the back the shoulders lying easily on the torso, the arms free, the sternum lifted.

- Finally allow the seven vertebrae of the neck to restack, the throat remains uninvolved, and last the head rebalances, floating atop the long neck and spine, the breath continuing to move the body from inside.

Title: Spinal zipper: Part 2

Aim: Deepening released alignment with partner facilitating.

- Partnering by twos: Partner A stands in front and partner B stands behind. Partner A stands well with feet parallel, shoulders down and wide.

- Partner A does a spinal zipper as partner B observes or rather witnesses – a witness is an interested participant – able to report and to testify fact and feeling without the need to criticize. Partner B gives minimal feedback – example: 'your neck was very released going down, but began to rise before the shoulders were finished and the clavicle in place on the restack'. Or 'I saw your belly move freely when you were fully released in the zipper.'

- A stands well and then B encourages A to release tension. Use words like 'release', 'let go', and a gentle touch to bring awareness to any held tension in the neck, head, shoulders, arms, upper and lower back, the upper chest, the upper belly, the lower belly, the alignment of the pelvis, the thighs, the knees, or the feet.

- B stands behind A and, beginning at the occipital joint of the head/neck with the balls of the fingers, gently circle on the vertebra to suggest that A release the head forward. B continues down the neck, pausing at the base of the neck to take the weight of the head in the cupped hands and gently lift then release it forward and down again.

- With the pads of the first two fingers giving guidance B circle on each vertebra of the back guiding release from the top of the thoracic vertebrae to the sacrum.

- Partner B continues to give gentle reminders to release the belly, arms, encouraging A to keep breathing, let the bones support the body, use minimal muscular involvement and maximal breath movement.

- Partner B places hands in a V shape (thumbs together fingers fanning out to the W) at the base of the ribs, fingers on the bulging side ribs and back of partner A. Partner B then gives enough pressure on the lower part of the rib accordion for A to feel the movement of breath in the lower back on a deep inhale.

- While dropped over, with shoulders released and head down, released knees, soft belly, the breath wants to move into the deep lungs, the low back of the body.

- B guides A into rolling backup one vertebra at a time until Partner A is standing upright.

- Partner A slowly opens eyes and takes a walk around the room, noting what may have changed, what feels longer, wider, more open, any places of tension and where the breath is travelling in the body.

- The partners switch roles and repeat the above. Having completed this both partners share observations of self and partner using phrases like 'I observed, I saw, I noticed, my body felt and my emotions were, etc.'

BIBLIOGRAPHY

Berry, Cecily (1998) *The Actor and the Text*. London: Virgin Books, New York: Applause Books Scribner.

Hackney, Peggy (2002) *Making Connections: Total Body Integration Through Bartenieff Fundamentals*. New York: Routledge.

Lessac, Arthur (1980) *The Use and Training of the Human Voice*. New York: Drama Publishers.

Linklaker, Kristin (1976) *Freeing the Natural Voice*. New York: Drama Publishers.

Rodenburg, Patsy (1993) *The Actor Speaks*. New York: St. Martin's Press.

Rodenburg, Patsy (1993) *The Need for Words*. London: Methnen Drama.

Rodenburg, Patsy (1993) *The Right to Speak*. New York: Theatre Art Books.

Rywerant, Yochanan (1983) *The Feldenkrais Method: Teaching by Handling*. San Francisco: Harper and Rowe.

Totton, Nick and Edmondson, Em (1988) (Online ed.) *Reichian Growth Work: Melting the Blocks to Life and Love*. Online: Prism Press.

CHAPTER 16

Laban and Breath

The embodied actor

KATYA BLOOM

In my work as a teacher of Laban-based movement at the Royal Academy of Dramatic Art (RADA), I am interested in facilitating actors' appreciation of the fact that the body, as well as the voice, can speak – that, in fact, the body is *always* speaking. I am interested in stimulating actors' recognition of what it is to be 'embodied'. Without embodiment, the actor is relegated to the realms of mental and imaginative processes only, without these necessarily being rooted in the here (of space) and the now (of time). Embodiment requires an awareness of and engagement with a sensitive and articulate three-dimensional body. One primary goal of this work is to explore the embodiment of psychological and emotional states in the actor's process of transformation. In this chapter, I will describe how the embodiment of the breath is also an implicit element in the working process.

BREATH AND THE DIALOGUE OF ACTIVE AND RECEPTIVE

If the exploration of movement is to be an involving and deeply-felt experience for the actor, that is, felt to have meaning beyond movement as exercise, then the actor must first recognize that moving with awareness, even in very simple and basic ways, such as stretching and yawning, changing positions and levels – from lying to sitting to crawling to standing and moving through space, etc. – not only feels good, but offers a gateway to releasing the breath and imagination, and expanding one's creative range and potential.

Moving in new ways can stimulate a sigh of relief, or a yawn of relaxation, a sharp intake of air, or a slow and measured exhale. Through connecting movement and breath, the mover can find release from unconscious patterns of holding the body up or holding oneself together in habitual ways. With release of breath and movement comes release of expression. With release of expression comes greater potential to feel and to think in new ways, to develop new experiences. In order to be someone other than themselves, actors need to be curious about challenging their own patterns, to explore the limitations of their presumed range.

One of the most essential elements in students' exploration of movement is learning how to relax their bodies and thereby allowing their movement to *breathe* and their breath to *move them*. As the body relaxes, so does the breathing; and, slowly, slowly, unconscious patterns of holding can begin to loosen and unclench. As implied already, these patterns are simultaneously physical, psychological and emotional. Receiving one's condition, which includes one's breathing, precedes expression. As students relax they can feel the support from the ground, from gravity and from the air around them; and they can allow the air to come in and go out.

The movement of the body is inherent in the act of breathing – breathing itself is movement and movement, if felt, 'breathes'. We can think of the whole organism breathing – the skin breathing, the feelings breathing, the mind breathing. The breath can anchor the actor's imagination in the here and now. It is my experience, however, that directly 'watching' or 'using' or 'contemplating' the breath, can often be counterproductive. It can set up an atmosphere in which there is a right and wrong way and the teacher is the authority. This can stifle creativity. I prefer a laboratory atmosphere of free exploration of themes, where good technique is discovered rather than imposed.

Through engaging in their own organic movement, the natural breathing will automatically be given space and time. They are not trying to fit their breath into a prescribed pattern, but rather, through developing their own movement vocabulary, to allow *breathing space* and freedom of expression. Different qualities of movement – faster, slower, bigger, smaller, longer, shorter, etc. – stimulate different qualities and rhythms of breath. I will expand on this when describing Laban movement analysis (LMA) in more detail.

The actor's art involves taking in and giving out; in this sense it could be conceived of as a breathing process. The taking in involves being receptive to both internal and external stimuli. The giving out involves active expression of need, desire and intention through voice and action. Through this exchange of active and receptive modes, through a dialogue of affecting and being affected, the actor communicates the complex panoply of forces of circumstance and emotion which are evoked by and contribute to the dramatic structure and atmosphere of a play. The inner dialogue – that is, what is going on within oneself – and the outer dialogue – what is going on between oneself and others – are often in conflict. It is the actor's job to embody this conflict between the private and the public with integrity. The signifiers of the complex elements of 'character' are inscribed in the physical body; and the character's breathing is an integral part of this bodily language.

Literally speaking, the breath mixes and exchanges what is outside and what is inside. It acts as a bridge between the two realms. On a more metaphorical level we could think of *breathing into consciousness* something which was not consciously known before. The breath might be thought of as a membrane separating conscious from unconscious. In the novel *Suite Française* by Irene Nemerovsky, in which the takeover of France by the German army in the Second World War is depicted, the author often describes the deep sighs that accompany characters' recognition of what is happening, the letting into consciousness what was previously defended against. Psychoanalyst Christopher Bollas coined the term 'the unthought known' to refer to that which is known but is below the level of conscious recognition (Bollas 1987). I wonder if assimilating and digesting the 'unthought known' depends upon the ability of both body and mind to open a space to receive it, to breathe it in – and to release or breathe out the mental and physical protections against knowing.

How does the actor practise movement?

Students are guided in a process of discovering *their own* movement vocabulary, based on working with specific themes. In this way they discover for themselves the depth of meaning evoked and conveyed through the nonverbal realm. They discover the way in which movement nourishes and fuels the emotional, psychological and imaginative processes, as well, of course, as enlivening and enlarging them physically. Exploring movement promotes an integrated experience for the actor of being inside the skin of others, rather than 'playing' a character but feeling somewhat separate from the experience. Articulation is a word that applies to both verbal and nonverbal communication. In my view both must be developed simultaneously in order for the actor to achieve full expression.

In my work at RADA, I draw on the language of Laban Movement Analysis (LMA) as the main source of inspiration. I use LMA to encourage the systematic exploration of a wide range of movement dynamics and states of mind, as well as the awareness of the body's relationship to and orientation in space. I also incorporate the approach of Indonesian movement artist, Suprapto Suryodarmo's Amerta movement, as a way of guiding students in a focused but non-stylized exploration of free movement, aimed at 'tuning' their bodily instrument.

For Suryodarmo, movement provides a 'bridge to understanding' and growth. Part of the challenge for students is to tolerate not knowing exactly what will emerge. By learning to trust the logic of what is unfolding in the moment, students learn to desist from prematurely making conscious decisions and foreclosing deep exploratory work. Suryodarmo speaks of finding safety through discovering the right proportion in relationship to space and time, not too big or too small or fast or slow to feel comfortable and present – this implies being *in* the breathing as well.

These two approaches, LMA and Amerta, most often blended together, support students in consciously recognizing their own qualities and strengths as well as their potentially limiting psycho-physical habits. The work increases their confidence and curiosity and broadens their range of expression. Both approaches are inherently connected to breathing, the focus of this volume, but perhaps their emphases and thus their effect on breath, differ. Broadly speaking, I would say that LMA is a more *active*, expressive, traditionally western approach; Amerta, a traditionally eastern approach, is more *receptive*. The balance of active and receptive is an important overall theme in the work and could be said to define the essence of what the art of acting requires.

My aim is to offer a palette of tools that will support students' ability to make their own *in-formed* creative choices. I ask students to follow the flow of their own internal logic in the movement, to find out for themselves what their bodies can and want to do. Through this approach, actors learn to make movement their own and fill it with breath. This approach supports actors' intention to spontaneously interact with fellow actors and with the environment. When they realize they are being invited to follow their own needs, they come alive; and breath, along with creativity, is released – into movement, sound and speech.

The guided explorations of movement vocabulary are often made within the context of research into the characters and plays students are working on in acting classes or projects. Students appreciate the freedom to discover from the perceptual perspective of their bodies and they repeatedly report that movement reveals insights about their characters which they would never have discovered through a conceptual analysis. It is one thing to know intellectually that there are conflicting parts of a character's personality, but it is quite another to experience these viscerally and explore the ramifications through movement.

This work makes clear the value Stanislavski placed on physical action, and in fact works hand-in-glove with a Stanislavski-based approach. LMA might help actors follow his guideline:

> Without forcing anything, carefully start from the simplest organic action. For the time being, do not think about the character. As a result of your correct actions in the given circumstances, the role, the character will appear. You don't have to play anything. (Toporov 1998, p. 131)

This approach is much more likely to draw on the unconscious and lead actors to make choices other than those in their habitual stockpile. If Stanislavski had known about LMA, I imagine he would have found it a highly complementary resource

LABAN MOVEMENT ANALYSIS (LMA)

Laban himself says this about movement,

> Movement is the result of the striving after an object deemed valuable, or of a state of mind. Its shapes and rhythms show the moving person's attitude in a particular situation. It can characterize momentary mood and reaction as well as constant features of personality. (Laban 1950, p. 2)

The system of movement analysis defined by dancer/choreographer/theorist Rudolf Laban from the 1920s until his death in 1958 and continually refined by his successors until the present day, holds great value in supporting actors' involvement in and appreciation of the nonverbal realm. Actors and directors increasingly recognize Laban's language of movement as a useful rehearsal tool. Used as a broad umbrella, LMA can provide structure for a wide variety of movement experiences, allowing for a freedom of exploration while at the same time providing a vocabulary with which to anchor and reflect on the experiences. By engaging in movement with a variety of different qualities, one's breathing is automatically released and engaged in different ways. I will try to illustrate this as we go along.

Effort theory

> The value of characterization through movement lies in the avoidance of the simple imitation of external movement peculiarities. Such imitation does not penetrate to the hidden recesses of man's inner effort. (Laban 1950, p. 20)

The Effort theory of LMA is a means for describing the relationship between movement and motivation. It defines, in movement terms, the components of psychological and emotional states. Laban delineates weight, space, time and flow as the four basic inherent qualities of movement. These four elements form the basis for an extended framework for describing, analysing and experiencing aspects of human behaviour.

From the starting point of the basic Effort qualities, one can embody a rich movement vocabulary and a complementary range of moods, actions and attitudes. For the actor, this yields creative fruit on many levels, not least being the recognition of one's own characteristic movement qualities; or, looked at another way, one's habitual patterns – physical, emotional and mental – as these inevitably shine forth in exploring the work. Such exploration also gives rise to specificity and clarity in one's choices, both in playing actions, as well as physical characteristics of character – body attitude, gestures, centre, tone of voice, ways of moving through space, facial expressions, activities, etc. Drawing on themes from LMA, actors discover that they can communicate as much with their movement as with their spoken words, that what they do, even in apparent stillness, can be as important and evocative as what they say.

By giving names to psycho-physical experiences, the vocabulary helps to elicit, contain and focus the actor's feelings. The LMA framework can provide the safety to risk going further afield than one might at first feel comfortable doing and can support actors in achieving a version of the same emotional state night after night. At the same time, they develop a sense of confidence and freedom to allow a performance to be fresh and live; as director Mike Alfreds puts it, to be, within given parameters, 'different every night' (Alfreds 2007).

The basic effort elements

The elements of weight, space, time and flow can be explored in terms of which ones predominate in an individual's or character's experience, which are the key motivators and how, depending on the given circumstances, the predominance may change. These elements can be linked with the natural elements of earth, air, fire and water respectively, which may help readers to sense and imagine how different qualities of breath are evoked simply by engaging with these basic categories. Laban also named two ends of a spectrum in terms of how each element is expressed and of course, this too affects the nature of the breath.

The element of weight relates to the physical-sensory world, the actual material substance of the body and the sense of touch. Think of the natural element of earth. The activation of weight requires an intention. Often this involves our intentions toward other people, who, in drama as in life, may or may not be receptive. The element of weight, then, is related to one's ability to have an impact, one's sense of agency. The use of weight is either *strong* (forceful) or *light* (gentle).

In terms of breathing, the reader can imagine, or try to explore, how, as one uses more physical force, the pressure becomes stronger, the air seems to become denser, the breath deepens and becomes more muscular to support the strong engagement. Contrariwise, if there is delicate use of one's weight, as in handling a teacup, the breathing becomes more rarified and both body and breath are experienced as finer, lighter. The element of weight evokes the visceral breathing of the body itself.

The element of space relates to one's perspective, one's point of view on the outside world. It implies a space for reflection and thought and is therefore related to the mind, to the mental aspect of experience. In natural elements, think air. The challenge for the actor is to embody the mind, so that he/she can be inside the story and not seeing or imagining it from a distance. The use of space is either *direct* (sharp focus) or *flexible* (broad overview). Try noticing the difference in your breathing when your focus is sharply direct, focused on the details in your environment, real or imagined; and notice how this differs from when, like looking thorough a picture window, you want to experience the overview, the entire landscape, rather than the details. The element of space evokes the breathing of the mind.

The experience of time – the rhythm, the impulse, the natural order of events and change – is an inherent and intuitive aspect of human experience. In natural element terms, think fire. Actors learn to sense the pulls toward past or future and discover how to be *in* time rather than only *on* time. Time is either *sudden* (accelerating) or *sustained* (decelerating). Notice the difference in breath when accelerating your movement and when slowing things down. Even the intention to speed up or slow down affects breath. The element of time evokes the breath of intuition.

Finally, the element of flow is associated with the *continuity* of movement, and implies a direct link with the relative freedom or restriction of the flow of breath and energy. This element has a bearing on the conscious or unconscious effort to control or release the flow of feelings and the experience of emotion. Of interest is how the flow of energy and feelings opens toward or closes away from relationship. Flow also speaks more practically of the degree of *precision* in movement. Flow is either *bound* (controlled) or *free* (abandoned). Imagine flow like the element of water – it either flows freely or its flow is measured or restricted in order to control the degree of flow. The element of flow evokes the emotional breath.

Of course these elements are not experienced in isolation, but rather in combination with each other. But in general, we can say that taken together, the physical, the mental, the intuitive and the emotional realms of human experience can all be awakened and charged through the movement practice. One student put its value to actors like this: 'Movement is not accidental, but has resonances deep in the psyche and emotional makeup. The vocabulary of Laban offers signposts as to where a character's journey will go, as they can signify a throughline of character development.'

Table 16.1 Basic Effort Elements

Quality	Association	Realm of experience stimulated
Weight (strong or light)	Intention	Physical sensation/ Impact
Space (direct or flexible)	Attention	Thought/Orientation/ Perspective
Time (sudden or sustained)	Decision	Intuition/Pace
Flow (bound or free)	Progression	Feelings/Control

Effort Actions

The Effort Actions describe the eight distinct possible ways of combining the elements of weight, space and time. In these very specific actions, the element of flow is in the background. The Effort Actions are named as follows: *punch, float, glide, slash, press, flick, wring, dab.* I like to work with these purely physically at first so that they are each embodied precisely and their distinct qualities can be perceived. For example, a punch is felt to be a strong use of the whole body, which arrives at a point in space and time, whereas a slash, which is also strong and sudden, never comes to a point, but trails off in space, producing an entirely different mental and emotional attitude. I do not wish to interpret the specific meaning of each of these actions because depending on the circumstances, a punch can be angry, joyful, determined, fearful, etc., as can a slash or any other Effort Action.

Physicalizing the effort actions leads quite organically into discovering a range of physical and breath rhythms and accompanying emotional states, gestures and postures. These actions can inspire an exaggeration of feelings, both those which are outwardly expressed and those which, for reasons both conscious and unconscious a character may be holding back from expressing – as mentioned earlier, the 'unthought known'. Working with the Effort Actions, actors can explore a broad range of choices in attitude and quality, which can reveal unexpected insights. These explorations will automatically dramatically affect the breathing.

Once actors engage with any of these actions fully in movement, the emotional and psychological effect lingers and they can then gauge the appropriate degree of intensity or subtlety in the outward colouring of expression, including how posture or gesture may be affected. An exploration of these actions helps actors discover how they believe a character will behave in order to further their objectives. Effort Actions can be especially interesting when used to characterize aspects of a person which may only be revealed in the slightest of shadow movements. The complexity of characters, the inner conflicts which are the stuff of drama, can be explored using the Effort Actions.

The Effort Actions can also be used in working with the voice, as sound and speech flow naturally from movement. With the actor's words, does she wish to press or float or wring to best achieve her objective? Embodying the Effort Actions helps to find the breath support for each specific choice. The Effort Actions can stimulate the imagination, acting as triggers for the actor to find the quality of voice and vocal rhythms of a character. They are also effective for trying out unlikely ways of expressing a character's thoughts and feelings. In playful exploration, kernels of unexpected authenticity can be revealed.

To experience how immediate the effect on breath is, try saying a line with each of the effort actions below. Try to physicalize the action first, making sure that you are involved in all three effort qualities at once. Once the action and the underlying breath and thought pattern are established, you can always tone it down; in fact, you can forget about the Effort Action. It has been a springboard.

Try playing an action toward a partner, for example, to annoy him or her. Try this by dabbing your words, then gliding, then pressing. Try an action of seducing your partner, using wringing, then floating, then flicking. Try these in the extreme at first, then find out how much is enough and which one(s) work best.

Table 16.2 Effort Actions

Action	Weight	Space	Time
Float →	Light	Flexible	Sustained
Punch →	Strong	Direct	Sudden
Glide →	Light	Direct	Sustained
Slash →	Strong	Flexible	Sudden
Wring →	Strong	Flexible	Sustained
Dab →	Light	Direct	Sudden
Flick →	Light	Flexible	Sudden
Press →	Strong	Direct	Sustained

States of mind and transformation drives

Effort theory goes on to define *states*, (which combine two basic effort qualities, and *drives* which, like the effort actions, combine three. These further expand Laban's analysis of the complexity of behaviour as defined by Effort qualities. He observed that two of the four basic elements are usually motivating a person at any time, while the other two, though present, remain in the background. These six combinations of two qualities each have a name which broadly describes a state of mind. For example a lazy stretch upon waking up would likely be classified as an example of *dream state* which involve a combination of weight and flow, the physical and emotional elements; its opposite state is called *awake state*, combining elements of time and space. It is an outwardly focused state of alertness and decision – the mental and intuitive aspects are activated. A spectator at a tennis match may characterize this alert state. The breathing of physical sensation and feeling in dream state will be different from the breathing of mind and intuition in awake state.

Transformation drives include three elements, one of which is flow, making them especially emotional. Like the Effort Actions, also motivated by three elements, they are the outward manifestation of the attitude expressed by a state. I have given a fuller description of States and Drives in previous writing (Bloom 2003, 2006). But for our purposes here, suffice it to say that, when fully embodied, the different states and drives naturally stimulate and are underpinned by their own particular rhythms and qualities of breathing.

Space Harmony

> 'the shapes of movement through space
> are always more or less coloured by a feel-
> ing or an idea. (Laban 1966, p. 48)

Space Harmony is the name for another area of Laban's work, which concerns the body's relationship to and orientation in the surrounding space. Without going into detail, I can suggest that the use of movement to explore such issues as orientation to space, the size of personal space, the body's shapes and gestures can all provide actors with a rich source for generating creative material when exploring a character or scene. Working with these themes will directly affect the quality, quantity and phrasing of breath, without needing to focus consciously on breathing.

Here are some examples: try experiencing your relationship to length, width and depth respectively; see how this alters your orientation to the space as well as your breathing. Imagine a small personal space and see how your breathing changes when you imagine a large space. Feel your relationship to particular points in the space, in front or back, above or below; notice if this stimulates your breath and if there are any emotional or imaginative resonances. Imagine where in your body you feel a character's centre to be and notice how your breathing automatically follows your mind.

SUMMARY

To summarize, LMA provides starting points for organic explorations in movement, through which the breath is naturally released and shaped in numerous ways. These starting points give actors the freedom to explore the depth and complexity of characters' experience and to contact the intentions and feelings which underlie, precede, prompt and colour a line of thought and choice of words.

I have observed that having a language of movement helps actors apply discipline to what is spontaneous. Using LMA as a framework, they can more easily awaken and trust their intuition in movement. It is my feeling that once the bodily experience is made conscious and integrated with the psyche, actors can then (and only then) fully experience the breath, the space, their relationships with each other, with the environment and the text.

Communication, on stage and off, does not only have to do with speaking; it also has to do with embodied presence, including, crucially, breathing. As audience members, we breathe in the emotional atmosphere of a play. The powerful transmission of atmosphere comes across when the actors are fully engaged in their own three-dimensional embodied experience. When this is the case, the body and its breathing can communicate directly, without going through a cognitive process. This communication, often of the most elemental of human feelings, does not depend on words; yet it has the potential to go right to the core of our being.

By providing a vocabulary with which to explore their range of motion and emotion, with an accompanying range of rhythms and qualities of breath, LMA is an invaluable tool for actors. By inspiring actors to embody their imaginations, LMA provides a springboard from which actors can breathe life into their characters.

BIBLIOGRAPHY

Alfreds, M. (2007) *Different Every Night: Freeing the Actor.* London: Nick Hern Books.

Bloom, K. (2003) 'Moving Actors: Laban movement analysis as the basis for a psychophysical movement practice'. *Contact Quarterly*, 28(3): 11–17.

Bloom, K. (2006) *The Embodied Self: movement and psychoanalysis.* London: Karnac.

Bollas, C. (1987) *The Shadow of the Object: Psychoanalysis of the Unthought Known*. London: Free Association.

Laban, R. (1950) *The Mastery of Movement*. London: Macdonald and Evans Ltd.

Laban, R. (1966) *The Language of Movement*. London: Macdonald and Evans Ltd.

Nemerovsky, I. (2006) *Suite Française*. London: Chatto and Windus.

Toporov, V. (1998) *Stanislavski in Rehearsal: The Final Years*. New York: Routledge.

CHAPTER 17

The Breath

Heart and soul of the self

JUDYLEE VIVIER

I am an actress. I am also a teacher of graduate acting students. But it is the particular lens of being an actress that has defined my journey both as artist and teacher. I am also a human being in search of inner peace, wisdom, discernment and knowledge about how to live this gift of life meaningfully. The common connection among these points of view is the breath and it is this relationship I would like to explore.

Breath is transformative. The craft of acting is not exclusively an art of breathing, but breathing is the basic action that supports the transformative art and craft of acting. Awareness of and connection to the breath, the release of excessive muscle action, which inhibits the breath and restricts the voice, is the essence of the craft I practise and teach. The action of breathing, the nucleus of the impulse, is the 'inspiration'. It is this impulse for the breath to enter and be received by the body, which is the moment of inspiration for action. It is from this place that student actors learn to work and create with honesty, vulnerability and power.

The impulse for the breath is the source of life: it reflects emotional, physical and intellectual states of being. It is the vital spirit, soul and mirror of all that happens between birth and death. Without full, deep, conscious and mindful breathing it is easy to disconnect from that vital essence that is the very source of life, consciousness and self. Breath is the fundamental element necessary to be an aware actor, teacher and human being.

Acting is all about transformation, but transformation from an authentic core. As such, there is an essential and personal connection to the spirit of 'the self' involved. The actor is the instrument through which the story is told and if the actor is unable to access his authentic self, or is fearful of what that process will open up, the work will not be truthful but instead will be veiled beneath the 'social mask' of what is acceptable, worthy of approval and predictable. So the ultimate goal of my practice is to encourage the actor to return to the breath. They must learn to 'listen and feel' with the entire instrument in order to liberate the self, to honour impulses, to release the natural voice and let go of individual tensions established by the need to defend, to protect, to mask vulnerability and emotional stirrings. The actor must be willing to expose, reveal and express the inner landscape through the breath, voice and body to avoid 'describing' thoughts and feelings through preconceived vocal and physical direction. Thus acting, the voice and the breath cannot be separated: the voice, the vibration of sound, is the external release of dynamic expression that rides on the outgoing breath revealing this innermost landscape.

Since acting is a craft essentially dependent on the breath impulse and release of physical holding patterns that block impulses, it is imperative to recognize the spiritual and physical transformative power of the breath that opens the vocal passage through which a fuller, more resonant, richer, more dynamically expressive voice can freely flow. With each year I practise my craft as an actor and a teacher, I become more convinced that this potential for transformation and true connection to self must be embarked upon with more directness in the training. How, then, do we train theatre artists to meet the demands of a changing theatre as it reflects our dynamic, ever shifting universe? The conclusion begins to take shape: we must teach an awareness of self and others, vulnerability, a willingness to risk not knowing, a sense of curiosity and passion. Imperative in actor training is the ability to undo excess holding in one's body, voice and thinking. In recent years it seems that students of all ages are increasingly reticent and defensive about real interaction, vulnerability, intimacy. They are unwilling and unable to leave themselves alone to reveal their honest thoughts and feelings. The development of the individual spirit and psyche, based on a more holistic healing process through the breath, is vital to voice and acting training: it is about bringing the self to the work.

My personal quest for continued growth as an artist is fundamental to my process as a teacher. I am a better teacher when I am involved in the creative process of acting and I am more specific as an actress when I am involved in the process of teaching. By actively practising my craft, physically and emotionally grappling with the creation of the character and her story, the exchange in the classroom becomes more meaningful, founded upon a richer 'living' understanding. This immediacy of participation allows more effective illumination of some of the more illusive quests in acting, such as:

- What does it mean to truly be present and in the moment?

- What does it mean to be in one's body instead of in one's head?

- How does one allow oneself to be vulnerable and what is the power of vulnerability?

- How does one trust oneself?

- How does one leave the self alone and be willing not to know what comes next?

- How does one 'own' the text?

- How does one 'fill' the space and the words so that the spoken word becomes a visceral experience?

Each of the above challenges is rooted in and related to the breath because they are linked to how we feel about ourselves. The breath describes the relationship we have with ourselves through the quality of its action and interaction with the body. The voice is the external expression and manifestation of the inner landscape. The voice is affected by, and connected to this relationship we have with ourselves, because it relies upon the outgoing breath as a power source. The departure and arrival place for voice production, for effective verbal and physical communication, is the breath, which reveals and reflects our most internal feelings, thoughts and attitudes consciously or unconsciously through the amount of release and restriction it carries.

I have heard that we come to teach what it is we most need to learn. I needed to excavate my 'self'. I had to understand who and what that was. I needed to accept my self for who I am and to trust that I am enough; that I am worthy of abundance in every aspect of my life.

I grew up in Apartheid South Africa, a society of extremes and contradictions. It is made up of many cultures most of which were denied integration and inclusion. Apartheid is an Afrikaans word that means 'apartness', 'separation', and the policy very simply was to encourage separate development. As a child of mixed heritage, an English-speaking mother and an Afrikaans-speaking father who became Anglicized, there was constant tension between the two families.

It was a society based on judgement, divisiveness, censorship and repression on every level. The totalitarian government policy of Apartheid encouraged a mass mentality. Individuals were dangerous; consequently development of the self did not play a central role in the white stoic Calvinistic tradition that formed my background. Free expression of emotion was discouraged. I applied the techniques I learned as a young actor to 'put on' characters, articulating my speech specifically and carefully, breathing as little as possible, pushing my small, strident voice through a tightly clenched throat in open-air auditoriums. Heaven forbid if an authentic emotion did somehow manage to escape. To acknowledge a true emotional connection on stage, or off, was selfish, dangerous, made others feel uncomfortable and carried the dreaded possibility of loss of control. So I learned to become a professional at holding my breath, making my body physically smaller by tightening my muscles and squashing all inner stirrings, thus keeping my 'self' a guarded secret, even from myself.

Ironically though, South Africa has a rich culture because of these very contradictions. It is a culture that loves stories. At a very young age I developed an ear for the dramatic. I learned this from my mother, my grandmother and my aunts who always had a story to share. I grew up listening to the radio with my grandmother who was my primary caregiver while my mother and father worked. We spent many hours a day listening to the daytime radio 'soap operas'. As an only child these stories and my books were my entertainment. The cadences, the resonance, the intake of the breath and subtle expressions created vivid worlds of people, places and events in my imagination.

I left South Africa in the early 1980s and came to the United States on a Fulbright Scholarship to study for a Master of Fine Arts in acting. The training I received, although strong, was inconsistent in terms of what was encouraged in the acting class. Although English is my first language, as a foreigner the challenge was to learn to interpret an emotional language completely different from my own. 'Off the wall' behaviour was encouraged in the acting class. The emotional behaviour of the students was manufactured, manipulated, not based in self-awareness and honesty. Many, including myself, considered risk to mean wild and uncontrollable behaviour. The impulses seemed to come from a mental decision rather than a true connection to self-knowledge. Much of the behaviour that resulted often put other students in real physical danger. There was a focus on ego, that seemed to over compensate for the lack of impulses grounded in true awareness, confidence and trust that come from self-knowledge. I was encouraged to be more aggressive; I learned to jump in and take a 'risk'; but in hindsight, this 'impulse' came more from my desire to be considered a better actor.

Sometime after graduation I found Chuck Jones who had devised a series of vocal warm-up exercises to bring conscious awareness through physical sensation of one's holding patterns, thereby permitting a release and a connection to the breath, to the emotional life and vibrated sound with focus and concentration benefits that support the entire process. The release allows more breath to enter the body, more space allowing more resonance and vibration; a 'state of readiness' emerges from which the character's action can be played with clarity, ease and specificity. Since inspiration or impulse lies with the in-breath, the physical connection to the breath in the body enables a true merging of the actor and the character. This particular approach to the work 'demystified' the integral relationship between breath, body awareness, release of tension and increase of resonant vibration, which permits the self to inform and permeate the character with authenticity.

Jones' work was not just about learning a 'vocal technique'. It had to do with the intimate conscious acknowledgment of what was actually taking place within my internal life. It allowed me to experience a concentrated connection to myself, an acceptance of whatever feeling was present as I breathed, without any thought to the next moment, free of muscle manipulation or need tied to the ego.

I learned to allow the breath to 'drop into the body', to be received by the body when need is present and subsequently to 'drop out of the body', when the in-breath is ready to be released, with a focus on the moment when the in-breath becomes the out-breath (see Chapter 13 by David Carey). I discovered the sensation of the outgoing breath 'supporting' or 'marrying' the vibration and felt that specific moment of union, the experience of the vibrated sound moving through the unblocked vocal channel to effect an action; a change in the outside world was extremely empowering. The sound and vibration that resulted offered a physical expression of a deep sense of my most inner self, transformed into a concrete and powerful force. The impact this process had on me was immense. I was ready to be 'uncovered'.

This process of excavating the self layer by layer, initiated by Chuck, deepened as I discovered Patsy Rodenburg's approach to vocal production and acting. The focus of Patsy's work is more connected to the text in terms of owning the language: the physicality of the sounds, accessing meaning through the experience of sounds, textures, qualities and structure of language by means of total acceptance and acknowledgement of the self.

I continued to work with Chuck for some years as an actress and a young teacher, continuing the process of 'mining the self', which has its root planted firmly in the action of the free breath. My acting improved and today I am more present as a human being in my relationship to the world, other people and needless to say, my self. I accept my vulnerability and the power that is embedded within that vulnerability. As an actress, I can leave myself alone and allow the text to act on me and transform me emotionally, psychologically and physically in my connection to the breath and language. A life long process, there is always more to learn and more treasure to mine and the deeper the treasure lies the greater the emotional pain can be.

Over the years, I have filtered Chuck and Patsy's work through my own sensibility and personality, and have made it my own. I recognize with much gratitude how immensely and powerfully these mentors have impacted both my life and my work. Patsy has also inspired my particular interest in the way women relate to their voices, especially women who perform in public.

As a result and in particular over the past four or five years, my teaching integrates the deeper focus on breath work in acting training as a consciously therapeutic process as well as a way into making peace with and embracing the self. In the graduate actors I teach about the need to negotiate what may be jamming the accessibility to truth, vulnerability and self-reliance. This involves confronting all the light and the dark of the heart and the spirit that is tapped into as the tensions that stifle and suppress emotions are felt and let go. The process takes courage. But the welcome outcome, potentially unsettling at first, is the awareness of the need and the entitlement to speak freely by connecting with the breath, harnessing the energy and transformative power of the breath, which in turn supports the physical voice, the metaphorical voice, freeing the body.

I ask my students to become conscious and present in the moment, aware, so as to release muscles in the body that do not need to be engaged, to consciously take more breath into the body, to let it drop into the belly, the pelvis. I ask them to stretch, to bring awareness to the neck, the throat and root of the tongue, the jaw, the shoulders, ribs and abdomen. And by leading them in this process I am by default going to have to cope with the outpouring of extremely personal and internal issues that will be unleashed (see Chapter 5 by Rebecca Cuthbertson-Lane). Sometimes there is transfer of feelings and attitudes towards parental and authority figures; but I do not think this should be avoided since this is the means to 'unjamming the pipes', so to speak. The integration of the body, the breath, the voice, the mind and the heart, are all inextricably linked to the psyche, the personality, environmental influences, all experiences that have shaped the individual in front of me.

The way in which I work is therapeutic. It is about owning oneself, embracing fully all aspects of the self, the physical, the emotional, the intellectual, the psyche, in order to approach and uncover the layers and masks that limit the light of the true self so that the work can connect more honestly, simply and truthfully. This process is not always comfortable and can often be disquieting, joyful, painful, but usually enlightening if the student is accepting and desirous of change. This is a process of developing physical awareness through simple centring, breathing, releasing and stretching exercises, checking in physically many times a day, journalling these discoveries regarding the physical manifestation of the subterranean psychological issues. This process of discovery is encouraging and affords them a degree of self-trust and self-reliance. It allows the individual a way to accept shifts little by little and to begin to apply them to the work intellectually at first and then to experience the sensation physically and emotionally.

I am not a psychologist; nor do I pretend to be one. I advise my students that there is great advantage in seeking personal counselling while they journey to release this strangle hold on the self. Work/craft issues are life issues. And so, creating a private support system for themselves in which they can safely analyse these life issues appropriately as they emerge in the work and is crucial to their progress. They begin to understand, accept and commit more willingly and deeply to working through the self via an instrument that is more flexible physically, emotionally and intellectually.

The questions I ask in the first class of the first semester are, 'What relationship do you have with your breath? What relationship do you have with your voice?' Most times the blank faces give away the fact that this has never occurred to them prior to this moment. Let alone the fact that these questions might bear some relation to their acting training. They all understand that without breath there is no life, but they take it for granted especially if they are fortunate enough not to suffer from asthma or allergic reactions. The first five to six weeks of the semester, then, examines the anatomy and physiology of the vocal instrument, a physical exploration, repeated practice of the vocal warm-up that directly addresses the psycho-physical connections of the process, resulting in discussion regarding tension and mind-body connections. We spend a lot of time breathing, developing a conscious awareness of the breath, a conscious awareness of how we breathe, the quality of the breath, the relationship between the breath and physical tension in the body, understanding how breath is the essence of all aspects of performance. It is the power source, the supply of energy for the making of sound and vibration. It is the means by which the emotional life is touched, awakened and fed into the vibrated sound or voice. Breath is the energy that frees the mental process of inspiration and conveys it into sound and meaning. It is life and is therefore the core of the self.

Intimate and personal work happens in the room; it is absolutely necessary for the students to trust one another and, more importantly, to trust me. I try to bring myself as fully to the work in the classroom as possible: by breathing and being open and present myself, by sharing personal experiences related directly to the work and to my own struggles as an actress, by being willing not to know all the answers. After working with many teachers, many methods of approach to voice production and acting, there is nothing really new in our work. The basic principles are definitive but there are many doors through which we can enter the same room. I am very committed to the practice of yoga and meditation in my personal quest for growth as an aware, present, grounded and sensitive human being and it is impacting all aspects of my teaching as well. I want to be an effective teacher and therefore need to be fully present at all times with myself, with the students, with an awareness of what I am asking them to explore.

Over time and with patience, the student develops physical awareness of the self and as a result they begin to make the connections between the psychic tensions and challenges that restrict the physical body. I ask that the students keep a journal regarding their observations and discoveries, to note if they were able to make the necessary adjustments and how, to describe specific sensations and/or feelings in relation to the holding and the releasing of breath and body. This exercise quickly increases and strengthens their ability to observe processes with heightened awareness. This is a practical part of the process: the consciousness of the self is the first step toward understanding the need for adjustment, the practice of adjustment develops as a result of this awareness.

Through floor work, individuals become aware of the moment, leaving themselves alone, observing their breathing and emotions. As they progress, they are asked to integrate this awareness and knowledge into every day life. It takes time; but the connections they begin to make are truly insightful and help them to realize when and how they can leave themselves alone, to be, to breathe, to release and how that affects the way they perceive the world. This awareness translates into skills that will support them both in their work and their everyday life as long as they want it.

I continue to practise this work both as an actress and a teacher; it remains my life's challenge to be self aware and conscious, to bring the full sum of me to each moment of my life. Though specific circumstances and surroundings change, the constant, the conduit, the heart and soul of the artist and the human being is my unwavering belief in connection to the breath.

EXERCISE

Title:	Breathing on the floor
Aim:	To experience deep breathing by releasing habitual physical tension.
How often:	Daily.
Where:	On any floor surface with a mat.

- Find a place to lie down on your yoga mat where you can stretch out. Lie down on your back with your feet on the floor and your knees pointing to the ceiling.

You can place an inch thick book below your head, at the base of your skull. Get comfortable and then come to a still place. Keep your eyes open if you can.

- Allow the spine to be long on the floor, think of little pockets of space between each vertebra, so they do not have the sensation of being scrunched or squished. Lift the head momentarily and feel the tremendous weight of it and then gently lower releasing the muscles in the back of the neck. Gently turn the head from side to side to check to see if the muscles are soft and not held.

- Now let the muscles of the face slide towards the floor, as you have a sense of giving into gravity. If your eyes are open, let whatever you are focusing on come to you, avoid 'seeing' it. Open the mouth so that the teeth are not clenched together and allow the jaw to drop down and back towards the floor. The tongue is lying like a small rug on the floor of the mouth. Make sure you are not consciously holding the mouth open.

- Bring your attention to your breath. Do not change anything. Is the breath shallow? Where is the breath in the body? Allow the breath to drop in and out of the body.

- As you breathe, allow the back of the rib cage on the floor to widen. Allow the shoulders to widen and drop onto the floor. Let the floor take your full body weight. Allow a little more space in your armpits and in the shoulder joint and allow the upper arms to extend out of that joint and lie heavy on the floor. Check to see if your elbows are soft. The forearms are resting on the floor and the backs of the hands are lying on the floor with palms facing the ceiling.

- Keep breathing. Notice if the breath is still where you noticed it last or has something changed or shifted without you making it happen? Can you feel the breath in the palms of your hands?

- Gently notice how you are feeling, physically. Then notice how you are feeling emotionally. Are you feeling any subtle feelings rising to the surface? Just notice them, let them be there and breathe, gently, allowing the breath to drop in and out of the body.

- Now bring your attention to your belly. Let all the muscles in your buttocks go. Allow the hipbones to soften and widen, letting the pelvis take up as much space as it requires. Let the small of the back widen and drop down towards the floor. Release the pelvic floor. Allow that whole area to release and see if you can feel the breath drop lower into the body without trying to make it happen.

- Bring your attention back to the breath. Trust that your body knows how to breathe and allow it to happen. Notice now if your feelings have shifted or if there are any other sensations in the body.

- Allow the thighs to soften and extend from the hips, the knees are soft and if you are struggling to balance the thighs let the knees rest gently against each other. Let the calf muscles go. Feel the feet on the floor. Feel the ankles and let them go, feel the soles of the feet on the floor, feel the toes and the joints in each toe. Can you feel the breath in the soles of your feet? Does the in-breath have a colour? And the out-breath, does it also have a colour? Are you aware of your heartbeat? Can you allow it to be and just listen to it and listen to the breath? How are you feeling? What is the quality of the mind? Can you bring your attention now to the breath again? Can you feel the rhythm of the breath?

- There are three phases to the breath: the in-breath, the out-breath and between the out-breath and the next in-breath there is a little respite. Notice that moment of rest. Is it quite short or is it quite noticeable? Can you allow that respite to take a little more time by allowing the in-breath to be received by the body when the body is ready for it? Allow each phase to take the time it needs. Allow the breath to lead while you observe.

- Now bring your attention to the moment when the in-breath changes direction and becomes the out-breath? Watch the moment when the in-breath is ready to be released in an out-breath. Notice if there are any feelings or sensations coming up. Notice if there is any anxiety creeping in as we watch the breath. And at the moment of the next in-breath becoming an out-breath, release an easy sigh on that out-breath. And again; and this time add some vibration to that sigh, keep it easy.

- Choose a piece of text and when you are ready, as the in-breath becomes the out-breath release the text supported by the out-breath. Repeat a few times and notice how this feels. When you are ready, let the text go. Stretch through the entire body, roll onto your right side and then into prayer pose and slowly roll up though the spine to standing. Make sure you do not hold your breath. Take a few moments to record your discoveries and questions in your journal.

BIBLIOGRAPHY

Jones, C. (2005) *Make Your Voice Heard: An Actor's Guide to Increased Dramatic Range Through Vocal Training.* Second Edition. New York: Backstage Books.

Rodenburg, P. (1992) *The Right to Speak: Working with the Voice.* New York: Routledge.

Contributors

Katya Bloom, PhD, is a teacher at the Royal Academy of Dramatic Art. She has written *The Embodied Self: movement and psychoanalysis* and co-authored *Moves: a sourcebook of ideas for body awareness and creative movement*. Katya is a Certified Movement Analyst from the Laban/Bartenieff Institute of Movement Studies.

Jane Boston is Senior Voice Practitioner and Head of Research and Staff Development at the Royal Academy of Dramatic Art in London. In her twenty-year teaching career she has worked as a voice teacher, acting teacher and director in a number of British educational institutions and theatres, including the National Youth Theatre of Great Britain and the Central School of Speech and Drama. Prior to teaching, Jane was a founder member of Siren Theatre Company as performer, musician, writer and director. Jane divides her time between work in London and home in Brighton, where she lives with her partner and their daughter Ella.

David Carey is currently a Senior Voice Tutor at the Royal Academy of Dramatic Art. He has worked within higher education and professional theatre, including four years at the RSC. He returned to the RSC in 2004 to coach productions of *Julius Caesar* and *Two Gentlemen of Verona*.

Rena Cook is Head of Voice at the University of Oklahoma School of Drama where she teaches voice, speech and dialects. In her twenty-year career, she has served as voice and dialect coach or director for over 200 shows. Rena holds an MA in voice studies from the Central School of Speech and Drama in London, an MFA in directing from the University of Oklahoma. She is Editor-in-Chief of the *Voice & Speech Review* and is a Board Member of the Voice and Speech Trainers Association.

Rebecca Cuthbertson-Lane is a voice and dialect coach, and holds an MA in Voice Studies from the Central School of Speech and Drama, a Bachelors Degree in Education, and an Honours Bachelor of Arts in English Literature. She has coached *Pistachio Stories*, *Beckett's Shorts*, and *Full Frontal Diva*.

Debbie Green is a lecturer in movement for actors at the Central School of Speech and Drama. Her work focuses on fundamental bodywork and form. Her approach is directed by the power 'in' the body; its presence and energy and what emerges is beauty, congruency and artistry within the work.

Yolanda D. Heman-Ackah, MD, is a laryngologist who specializes in professional voice care. She received her Doctor of Medicine degree from Northwestern University and is Head of The Voice Center, Head and Neck Institute at the Cleveland Clinic, Cleveland, Ohio.

Kristin Linklater, the distinguished international voice practitioner, is a Professor of Theatre Arts at Columbia University, and originally trained at LAMDA. Her book, *Freeing the Natural Voice*, first published in 1976 and again in 2006, has been translated into seven different languages. Her second book, *Freeing Shakespeare's Voice: An Actor's Guide to Talking the Text*, was published in 1992.

Stephanie Martin, PhD, is a Speech and Language Therapist in London and a Past-President of the British Voice Association. Her career has combined clinical practice, research, lecturing and writing. Her most recent publications are: *The Teaching Voice*, second edition; and *VIP: The Voice Impact Profile*.

Tara McAllister-Viel is a Voice lecturer at the Central School of Speech and Drama. She received her PhD – Performance Practice in Voice from the University of Exeter, School of Performance Arts, England. She has been a professional Equity actress, voice-over specialist, Voice coach and director for the past eighteen years.

Marj McDaid's classical training in singing with Veronica Dunne and performance in improvised music fired her fascination with the voice. Exploratory workshops culminated in obtaining the PGDVS at the Central School of Speech and Drama in 1993. Marj works in the School of Acting at Arts Ed and is a freelance coach.

Michael Morgan has taught voice and speech at Yale School of Drama and the Theatre Conservatorium in Brussels. Michael is a designated Linklater teacher and a Fitzmaurice Associate teacher. He is a graduate of NYU, holds a MS from Samra University of Oriental Medicine and a PhD from UCSB.

April Pierrot, M'STAT, has been a senior tutor in Alexander Technique at the Royal Academy of Dramatic Art since 1992. Originally trained as a journalist at Carleton University in Ottawa, Canada, she worked for many years to the BBC World Service, before leaving to pursue her interest in Alexander Technique in 1986. She qualified as a Five Element Shiatsu practitioner in Dublin in 2001, and currently practises in London and elsewhere. For 20 years she has had a Yoga practice and trained with Body Primo in London. Her long standing interest in bodywork and bodywork systems has informed her interest in matters of skeletal alignment and functional anatomy.

Judylee Vivier is the director of the MFA acting program at Brooklyn College. She received an MFA from the Tisch School of the Arts and an MA and BA from the University of Natal, Durban, South Africa. Brooklyn College honoured her with the Claire Tow Award for Distinguished Teacher.

Joanna Weir Ouston is a Voice Coach, Theatre Director and Management Development consultant of international repute. She heads the Voice Department at Oxford School of Drama, lectures on the MA in Voice Studies at the Central School of Speech and Drama (London) and coaches professional actors and presenters.

Lisa Wilson is Professor and Chair of the Department of Theatre at the University of Tulsa. Her training comes from the University of Wisconsin, Madison MFA, BFA The University of Memphis. She is a Kendall College of Arts and Sciences Teaching Fellow and has received the University of Tulsa Outstanding Teaching Award. Mother of two sons and wife of a very patient technical director/designer.

Jessica Wolf trained as an Alexander Technique teacher in New York at the American Center for the Alexander Technique and was certified in 1977. In 1998, Jessica joined the faculty of the Yale School of Drama.

Index